BEING WELL

Beginning the Journey

of

Integral Lifework

T.Collins Logan

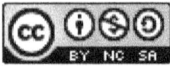

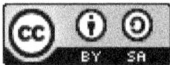

First Edition, May 5, 2012
ISBN 0-9770336-1-9

Published by the Integral Lifework Center
PO Box 221082
San Diego, CA 92192
www.integrallifework.com

For You

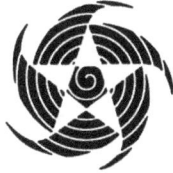

OTHER BOOKS BY T.COLLINS LOGAN

Memory: Self

True Love: Integral Lifework Theory & Practice

Essential Mysticism

The Vital Mystic: A Guide to Emotional Strength & Spiritual Enrichment

A Progressive's Guide to the New Testament

Please also visit www.integrallifework.com for articles, updates, discussion and additional information about the work of T.Collins Logan.

Special Thanks

Special thanks to my sister Karin for her feedback on my previous writing; not only was that feedback helpful in itself, but it became part of the inspiration to write this book. Thanks also to Oni, who provided input and edits on early drafts of *Being Well*. Special thanks to Elizabeth, whose critiques of my previous writing helped me appreciate simplicity. To Bill and Lori, much heartfelt gratitude for your excellent ideas about publicizing my writing. Bill also provided superb feedback on the final draft of this book, and challenged me to both expand my thinking and focus my language in much needed ways. And thank you to Pamela and Mollie as well for additional insights on the editing and review process.

TABLE OF CONTENTS

"In a beginner's mind there are many possibilities..."

– Shunryu Suzuki

FOREWORD

What does it really mean to "be well?" It probably depends on whom you ask. One kind of wellness is physical health, strength and vitality – some people decide that, if as person has lots of physical energy, and doesn't feel weak or exhausted from illness, this means they are well. Other people view wellness more in terms of what is happening inside the mind. For example, if a person is having mostly positive thoughts and making decisions that generally benefit their life, then they are considered mentally well. Another way to define wellness is through a person's overall happiness. Do they feel happy and content most of the time, or are they sad or angry? In this case well-being is defined more by the state of the heart. Other folks might measure well-being by the quality of personal friendships, romantic relationships or family relationships. For them, being well cannot happen unless there is harmony, kindness and satisfaction in these interpersonal relationships. Then there are those who focus on spiritual matters, who consider the state of a person's spirit or soul as the most important aspect of being well. And lastly there are people who view personal achievement as the most important measure of happiness. For example, is a person being productive with their time and reaching the goals they have set for themselves? If so, the satisfaction of their *doing* well becomes a measurement of their *being* well.

So there are really many different ways of looking at being well, each of them emphasizing different aspects of life: physical well-being, mental well-being, emotional well-being and so on. But why should we keep all of these different kinds of well-being separate? Why not look at the whole picture? In this book, we will explore how these different aspects of self can be combined into an overall sense of wholeness and completeness. We will see that, when each area cooperates and harmonizes with every other, "being well" really means growing and thriving in new and unexpected ways – combining, balancing and even transcending all of these dimensions. There is physical health, emotional health, spiritual health, healthy relationship, having a healthy purpose, and so on. But the most exciting discovery of all is observing how all of these different kinds of well-being work together to create something greater. It may just be a greater sense of contentment. Or it may be a greater kind of healing. Maybe even a greater personal transformation, or a greater influence on the world around us.

This approach to being well is based on the theory of Integral Lifework, which was developed over many years of interaction with my clients and students. Integral Lifework is about a simple, straightforward way to care for ourselves, others and the world around us. By providing balanced and harmonious nourishment for every aspect of our being, Integral Lifework helps us develop the awareness, compassion and skills to thrive and grow as a whole person. The process begins within you, and it quickly expands outwards to encompass everyone and everything around you as well. Given time, and with persistence and careful attention, Integral Lifework becomes an irresistible and far-reaching force of positive transformation.

I am hopeful that everyone – of any age, from any cultural background – will benefit from this book, spending time with these ideas and trying them out in practice. For the sooner anyone gets started down a path to wholeness and harmony, the sooner they can arrive at some truly amazing places. We all have tremendous potential within us, and Integral Lifework offers a powerful and rapid way to activate that potential here and now. It all begins by practicing a little essential self-nourishment each and every day. And the more people who practice this, both individually and in community, the more quickly and confidently we can achieve our own personal goals, and join together to meet the many challenges humanity must face.

A Whole Person Cares for Many Selves

The journey to wellness is a journey toward wholeness. Why? Because wholeness means encouraging harmony within ourselves, and trying to live in harmony with the world around us. When we aren't encouraging harmony, then all of our many needs and wants end up competing with each other for our attention. Our heart won't listen to our mind, our mind won't listen to our body, our spirit won't listen to our heart, and so on. Each of them is trying to go a separate way. Sometimes these inner impulses can even sabotage each other or cancel each other out. This is how we end up divided against ourselves, and this division increases our suffering. So every person is really made up of countless puzzle pieces, an infinite number of components, patterns and interactions. But in a *whole* person, all of these are working in harmony together. We can begin our journey towards wholeness by understanding all these different inner wants and needs, and helping them work together instead of against each other.

To help make that multifaceted inner world more manageable, Integral Lifework divides our being into twelve definable parts. Each of these parts represents a distinct personality, a unique identity with its own appetites and yearnings. So each of us really has twelve selves living within. These twelve selves are always changing and evolving – they aren't fixed identities carved from stone. In fact we could say they are more like children of all different ages, a whole family of selves. Some of them grow up quickly and become strong and mature, and others are still just starting out, still finding their way. Some have become confident and assertive, able to get their needs met easily, while others struggle more, lack confidence, or aren't sure how to get their needs met at all.   And just like flesh-and-blood children, these inner children require a lot of attention. They need to be encouraged and comforted. They need to be kept warm, get enough to eat, and be protected from the storms of life. They need to feel safe and secure and loved. They need to be listened to and appreciated. They need to feel like they have some power over their own existence – some control over what happens to them. And, just like any other children, they need to feel like they have freedom, too – freedom to explore, invent, experiment and learn.

So the main goal of this book is to help you identify and nurture twelve inner children. Because when your inner kids are well-cared-for, you will feel more complete, balanced and whole. And as you increase your inner harmony, all sorts of positive things begin to happen. You will experience more energy and less stress. You will feel healthier and happier. You will have a clearer sense of confidence and purpose. You will help prevent all sorts of physical illness and even heal existing illnesses. Your emotional life and your relationships with others will be enriched. You will enhance your mental clarity, creativity and insight. You will expand all of your senses, including your spiritual and intuitive awareness. You will overcome barriers you have experienced in the past, transform your own life, and discover new ways to be a positive, compassionate presence to others.

So whose responsibility do you think it is to care for our inner selves? Who is the real parent of our inner family? Sometimes we might conclude that others should be caring for our inner kids. Perhaps we think someone in our biological family should provide that care – our own parents, a sibling, or even a kind and caring relative. Or perhaps we think a few of our closest friends should bear the responsibility. Maybe we believe our girlfriend, boyfriend or spouse should have an important role in parenting our inner family. Or maybe a doctor, therapist or alternative health practitioner is supposed to help us nurture them. Perhaps we feel a spiritual teacher should provide us with guidance and advice. We may look to our work environment, neighborhood, community or government organizations for support. We might even be persuaded that a commercial product or service will somehow meet all the needs of our inner kids. And some people expect their own biological children – or even a beloved pet – to take some responsibility for this nurturing as well.

Do you notice the pattern here? All of these caretakers are outside of ourselves. They are not us, they are someone or something external to our innermost being. But why would we ever want someone or something outside of us to care for our innermost selves? Imagine if your own parents had always relied on other people to take care of you when you were a young child. That wouldn't be very good parenting, would it? Even if parents can find the very best, most skilled people in the world to raise their children, it will be hard for those children to feel fully loved and appreciated if their parents are never around – never expressing that caring or support directly and personally, never hugging their kids or laughing with them, never listening to their children's needs or spending time with them. In the same way, when we decide that someone else outside of us should care for our inner children, we aren't being very good parents, either. We are giving our most important responsibility away, and unintentionally showing those inner children that we don't really love them enough to engage them one-on-one.

Now this is a very important point, because we develop much of our identity – much of our self-concept – from interactions with our own parents. Kids will carefully watch how their parents interact with each other and the world to figure out how best to navigate new situations. So if our parents didn't demonstrate affection towards us when we were little, we may have difficulty giving and receiving affection as we grow older. If our parents always treated us as if we were stupid or incompetent, then we may conclude that we are in fact stupid or incompetent, or we may have a lot of insecurity and defensiveness around certain things. If we have seen our parents fighting all the time, or witnessed them feeling helpless and abused by the world, then we may grow up fighting with our loved ones or feeling like victims. On the other hand, if our parents were fully engaged with us in loving and skillful ways, and were able to model contentment in life and demonstrate successful interactions with others, then we will tend to grow up with a more positive, confident view of ourselves, and we will adopt more successful ways to interact with the world. So, in the same way, we need to become models for our own inner children. Rather than giving up all our skillfulness, nurturing and influence to others, we need to become skillful parents to our inner family.

There are many reasons why we look outside of ourselves for someone or something to care for our inner selves. It might be because we live in a commercialistic system with lots of advertisements, where we are constantly sold the idea that some product or service will improve our health, well-being and happiness. Or it may be what we learned from our peers or from our community that we are supposed to rely on them for nourishment – that in fact it is a suspicious or betraying act to become self-sufficient in certain areas. Maybe becoming overly reliant on people or things outside of ourselves was deeply ingrained in us through books, music, movies or other media we absorbed at a young age. There are many ways we can arrive at such self-limiting beliefs. But regardless of how we came to be dependent on external caretakers, we can't blame that dependence entirely on our biological family, culture or any other external sources. For that is just another way of not taking full responsibility for our own well-being and happiness. It is our choice in each and every moment to steer the direction of our life with our own efforts. And if we have been letting other people steer – or have been blaming them for leading us off-course – then we must learn how to let go of the impulse to externalize our well-being, and become more independent and self-sufficient. We must begin to look within ourselves for strength, courage and self-reliance.

At the same time, most of us do not live in isolation, but rely on each other to survive. Human infants are the most helpless of any species on Earth, completely dependent on their parents in the earliest years of life. As we grow up, we continue to rely on our family to support and guide us. As adults, we count on our family and friends for encouragement, wisdom, and help us in times of need. We rely on the people in our community to follow our society's rule of law, so we can all feel safe. We rely on public servants like firefighters and police officers to intervene whenever there is an emergency. We rely on our nation's military to defend us from foreign invasion. And we, in turn, provide material support, emotional encouragement and other assistance to others we care about. So in this sense self-reliance does not mean isolation from others, or rejecting participation in family, community or society. But it does mean that our first reflex is to look within ourselves for strength, insight and resources, rather than always looking somewhere else.

Through Integral Lifework we can become our own most trusted advisor, our own skillful guide in an unpredictable world, our own loving and patient parent.　And even then, the Integral Lifework approach itself is not really the answer, either.　It just provides some helpful hints and resources.　For all anything or anyone outside of us can do is offer some tips and tools for our journey, and a few road signs along the way.　So it is this orientation of self-trust that sets the scene for the rest of this book:　the pages that follow will offer encouragement to seek your own unique path, and the most powerful discoveries, strengths and answers will come from that journey within.　To begin, we will try to understand who each of our twelve inner children are, what they might need, and different ways we can provide for them.

Caring for Twelve Hungry Kids

As anyone who has spent time around large groups of children knows, just trying to oversee twelve children in any situation can be a daunting task.　It is easy to look at them as one big herd, running around, yelling, laughing, leaping and wrestling over toys.　But really we need to get to know each one individually, and interact with each one individually. We need to get a feel for who each child is, how they like to interact, their favorite activities and so on.　And the better we get to know each one, the easier it will be to care for them all.　It might be natural for us to favor one child over another, and to accidentally nurture our favorite children much more than the others.　But in order to care for our whole self, we need to find ways of balancing how we care for all of our inner children.　We need to prevent our natural favoritism from depriving or punishing the rest of our inner family without our even realizing it.　We need to become a fair parent.

Why is this so important?　Well, remember that each inner child may be at a different stage of development and growth.　Like any diverse group of kids, each one is likely to have their own unique gifts and strengths, and their own unique challenges to face.　This means that each child will naturally progress at their own pace, and may need special help with barriers to thriving that our other kids don't. So if we can't balance our attention between all our kids, some may get either so far ahead of the others that they demand all of our attention to remain content, or so far behind all of the others that they demand all of our attention to survive at all. I'm sure you've met people who are really smart but socially awkward; or people who are highly driven to succeed in their profession, but never exercise their body; or people who are artistically talented but clueless at math; or folks who might be charismatic and get along well with everyone, but who can't seem to follow through on anything they plan or say they will do. In other words, there are people everywhere who are out-of-balance because one part of them has been fully and continually nurtured, and other parts have not. It is a normal tendency for humans to become out-of-balance like this, because we like to gravitate to where our strengths are, and avoid our weaknesses. But doing this doesn't help us heal or grow in the areas that are essential to our well-being. We may always depend on our natural strengths to some degree, but if we remain too far out-of-balance, will are likely to become sick or unhappy…and we will never become whole.

In the following chapters, we will try to get to know each child, each inner self, one by one. First we will give each inner family member distinct names and personalities that are easy to differentiate and remember. That way, we can remind ourselves each day to nurture all of them. The names have been chosen from different cultures, each with a meaning that relates to the dimension of self that inner child represents, in the hope that this will add interesting flavor to our self-parenting experiment.

In each chapter, we will explore different ways of communicating with a particular inner child. Sometimes these techniques may seem strange or different – for example, visualizing an inner child and imagining we are having a conversation with them – but using our imagination in this way is a powerful tool. The relationships we create with our inner kids within our imagination allow us to develop strong bonds with every part of our inner life. However, like many things that are new and different, the real benefits will only become clear after practicing the techniques in this book for a while. As much as we might want to have instant and easy communication with someone, it sometimes takes effort, careful listening and many questions to fully appreciate and understand them.

Even when that person is part of our inner family – an aspect of our own being – we still need to be skillful, careful and patient as we get to know them more completely.

Questions for Reflection & Discussion

- Without yet having read the following chapters, what are some of the inner children – your dimensions of self – that you have already come to identify, or that you imagine might exist within you?

- What benefits do you think there might be in taking responsibility for caring for our own inner children, rather than giving that responsibility to someone else?

- Is it sometimes necessary to share responsibility for our self-care with others? If so, when? Whom can you trust to help you with this, without giving away too much responsibility?

- How did your parents nurture you when you were little? Can you see any evidence that their attitudes towards you – towards how you dress, for example, or towards your personality and behaviors – have had a lasting effect on how you view yourself, or how you view different facets of your personality?

- Do you believe you already have strength, courage and self-reliance within yourself? Why or why not? What are some recent experiences that demonstrate your levels of each?

- Would you say that you care for yourself in a balanced way? Why or why not?

- What attracted you to reading this book, and what would you like it to accomplish by reading it?

WONDERFUL WACHIWI – FOR A HEALTHY BODY

"Wachiwi" (wah-chee-wee) is a Sioux name that means dancer or dancing girl, and for me it describes the perfect attitude and expression of physical health. Why? Because physical health tends to involve lots of joy and pleasure, while at the same time demanding strenuous effort. Like dancing, it is as much an expression of life as a strengthening of our physical being. When we care for our physical selves, it can be as rewarding and fun as it is challenging or difficult.

Inside all of us, then, is a little girl named Wachiwi, and what she most wants to do is dance through life. When you bring her to a park, she yearns to run and skip and jump and twirl. When she finds herself sitting in an uncomfortable chair in a dimly lit room, all she can think about is getting out of that chair and running around. When she sees a tree, she wants to climb it. As soon as she wakes up in the morning, she throws off the sheets in eager anticipation of another day of joyful physical effort. When you bring her to a party, she can't wait to find someone to run, dance and play with her. Although she might be shy or hesitant sometimes, she just can't help herself: she always wants to be in motion. She loves to move her body, to feel the wind rush through her hair and across her sweaty skin. For Wachiwi, every muscle is like an itch to be scratched, a symphony of sound that longs to spring forth into rigorous action. At the end of the day, unless her limbs are sore and her chest raw from gulping breaths, she just doesn't believe she has had any fun at all.

However, not everyone believes they have Wachiwi inside them. Perhaps they can't hear her eager pleas to dance, or maybe they are embarrassed about how Wachiwi wants to make their body behave. Not everyone is a graceful dancer, after all. And not everyone can climb trees or skip rope or run fast. Not everyone can feel the joy of physical activity or the carefree satisfaction and release of skipping around a playground. It may also be that something in our culture or someone in our immediate family has told us that prancing about like Wachiwi wants us to is unseemly, impolite or unacceptable. And sometimes, if we are busy doing lots of other things throughout the day – things we believe are more important and which we aren't supposed to neglect – then making time to dance, run and play seems like a luxury we can't afford. And so for these reasons (or perhaps some other one), sometimes Wachiwi is left alone in a dimly lit room and totally ignored. Sometimes we even tell her to be still and quiet when she starts to make a fuss. And when this happens, it makes her very sad.

As with our other inner children, one of the most important parts of taking care of Wachiwi is just letting her be herself. To let her dance the way she longs to dance. To let her run around gleefully, getting all sweaty and dirty. Maybe she will accidentally ruin her nice clothes. Maybe others will look at her strangely. She might even stub her toe, or scrape her knee, or twist her ankle. But none of this really matters, because Wachiwi is doing what she most yearns to do, what she thinks about in every moment. And by allowing her to express her essence, we are showing Wachiwi that we love her and want her to be happy.

Now as her parent, we do have other responsibilities as well. For instance, we wouldn't want her to become seriously hurt, so we make sure she doesn't dance on the edge of busy highways or on a slippery rooftop or some other risky place. Everyone has different skills and a different level of confidence in each situation, so what is risky for one person may be easy and fun for another. Which means it takes time to figure out what is safe for our Wachiwi to do, and what is dangerous, and that this safety zone will probably change and evolve over time as well. All of this often takes a lot of trial and error to figure out, so that means Wachiwi needs as much freedom as we can provide her to explore the world – freedom to figure out where she can safely dance and skip and jump and run.

Another responsibility we have as Wachiwi's parent is to make sure she gets the rest she needs. Like many children, Wachiwi may not always want to go to sleep at night. She may want to stay awake. She may be afraid of the dark, or afraid of missing something exciting that could be happening. She may be cranky and tearful because we ask her to sleep. She may be insistent and stubborn about staying up as late as she wants. But what Wachiwi sometimes forgets is that when she is tired from lack of sleep, she doesn't have the energy to dance. Her limbs are sluggish and awkward. Her balance is off. She is more likely to injure herself doing the simplest things. And so, like any good parent, we gently explain this to her and help her find her way into a deep and satisfying rest. Then, in the morning, we help her get up at the same time each day, so that she can enjoy it to the fullest.

And of course Wachiwi needs to eat well and drink lots of water to have energy for dancing as well. She might be craving sugar, or fat, or salt or even caffeinated drinks...but as her parent you know better. Junk food may taste great at first, but afterwards we may feel sick or lethargic. Our skin may get oily and smell funny. We may have trouble sleeping or concentrating. And we are much more likely to gain unhealthy amounts of fat all over our body. The pleasurable rush that comes with satisfying these cravings may be exciting and even intoxicating at first, but it doesn't compare to the longer term and much deeper satisfaction of healthy food, unsweetened drinks and regular exercise. To eat well is to fuel the body for a purpose, and in Wachiwi's case that purpose is to be vigorously and joyously active every single day. Now there may be times that Wachiwi needs special things to keep herself strong, quick, agile and flexible, and so some of her cravings may actually communicate those needs to us. Maybe a hankering for ice cream reflects her need for some extra calcium; maybe her desire for potatoes is driven by a need for potassium; and maybe her appetite for bright red fruit indicates a need for Vitamin C; and so on. Listening to those cravings can therefore help us identify healthy things we can provide to help her be completely and lovingly nourished.

Now it is important to remember that when Wachiwi has been neglected for long periods of time, none of these things will come naturally or easily. She will tend to be lethargic and unresponsive, having forgotten many of her body's joys. She may even resist new routines and throw a tantrum or two. For if Wachiwi has been left alone too long in a dimly lit room, she will begin to believe that no one cares about her. That no one loves her. Just saying "I love you, Wachiwi, and I care," can go a long way to helping her feel less alone and less afraid, but as her parent you may have to demonstrate that love with actions over and over until she begins to believe you. For example, making a special place and space for her every day, taking her outside for long walks, giving her permission to be silly and free, showing her that you are willing to be embarrassed in public, so that she can be less afraid to express her nature.

It is also important to remember that becoming frustrated or angry with Wachiwi won't help very much, because if she hasn't danced in a long while, she really may not believe she can dance anymore. She may not think she can be strong, quick or graceful ever again. So as part of providing a good example, you may need to show courage and resolve and self-discipline. To say, "See, I'm trying to let go of my fears and inhibitions, and I'm trying to become stronger and quicker and more graceful every day. I'm doing this so that you can be your true self, and not be afraid anymore." Such valiant efforts are part of what truly loving our inner children looks like.

One last thing to think about is that our bodies are also connected to wilderness and Nature, and to the cycles of the moon, sun, planets and even the galaxy itself. Wachiwi knows when the moon is bright outside, and she loves to be taken out into that silvery light. She knows when Spring is coming, and wants to see the wildflowers blooming and smell their happy greeting. She senses the turnings of the year, when nights will be getting longer or shorter, and the days will become warmer or cooler. And she wants us to acknowledge those things, even if it is in small ways, because they are important to her. She wants us to pay attention. She says, "Look, the stars are different tonight!" Or "It's raining really hard!" Or "Doesn't the air smell like falling leaves right now?" Always, Wachiwi wants to dance, but just like the seasons and the phases of the moon, her moods – and the style, flavor and speed of her movement – change constantly.

Conversations with Wachiwi

Now to better understand what Wachiwi yearns for, we will need to have regular conversations with her. Most of the time, this means making sure she knows that she can tell us whatever is on her mind and heart, and listening to her as carefully and attentively as we can. If Wachiwi believes we care about her, and trusts that we are hearing what she is trying to say, and that we aren't intent on correcting her or persuading her to feel differently than she does, then she will be honest and open with us. If she trusts us, we will learn everything we need to know about Wachiwi and her world. Depending on the kind of relationship we have had with her so far in life, that trust may already be there...or we may have to rebuild it slowly over time.

All of this happens through open and honest dialogue, and so that is what we must begin to do, and what we must continue doing. There are many ways to have a conversation with Wachiwi, so I'll offer a few of them here to get you started. Maybe you already know some of them, and that's great. The key to all of these conversations is a quality of openness and sincerity in heart and mind. For example, let's say you are sitting next to someone while you wait for an appointment. They turn to you with a blank expression and ask, "How are you today?" But as soon as they ask, they look away or start talking to someone else, and you get the feeling that they are just asking you out of habit. This sort of empty interaction is the opposite of openness and sincerity, and we won't be able to have a real conversation with Wachiwi if we approach her this way. We have to be genuinely interested, to really want to know. Have you ever had a close friend you haven't seen for a while come running up to you and say, "It's so good to see you! How have you been? What's new in your life?" All the while, they hold your eyes in theirs, eager to understand what is important to you in this moment, and to share their experiences with you as well. This is the spirit of conversation that will help us get to know the innermost hopes and yearnings of all our inner kids.

So take a moment to sit somewhere that is quiet where you won't be disturbed, and close your eyes. Just sit comfortably with your hands resting lightly on your knees. Breathe slowly, deeply and evenly – through your nose if you can. Fold both hands over the lower middle of your chest, right where your rib cage ends and your stomach begins. Focus all of your attention on the space beneath your hands. Feel the pressure of your hands against your body, and the warmth that builds there as you hold your hands in place. Rest in that warmth and pressure for a while, continuing to breathe deeply, slowly and evenly. After a few minutes, and without opening your eyes, let your attention expand out from the center of your chest down into the pit of your stomach. Begin to feel around your stomach for any and all sensations. Is there heat anywhere? Or coolness? Is there a sense of fullness? Or of emptiness? Is there any firmness or tension? Any softness or relaxation? Can you hear any sounds or feel any sort of vibration? Are there any other qualities you can feel, like pleasure or discomfort? Spend a few minutes with your awareness resting in your stomach, and listen openly and sincerely for anything it wants to share. When you feel you have heard everything your stomach has to say today, open your eyes.

Once you feel comfortable with this exercise, try it each day with different areas of your body. You will want to always begin the same way, with hands folded over the lower middle of your chest, eyes closed, breathing deeply, slowly and evenly, with your focus centered on the place beneath your hands. Then shift your attention to a new part of your physical self. What does your foot have to say? Or your hand? What does your neck want to share with you? What about your lower back, or your kidneys? The muscles around your jaw? How about your eyes, knees or neck? You can pick any part of your body – if you can, try to focus some attention on each and every one over time. All of them are Wachiwi, and all of them probably have something to share with you.

Now if you have any difficulty hearing or feeling anything for a particular area of your body, there are other things you can try. For instance, you can say silently to one part "I just want you to know I really care about you and want you to be happy and whole. I am listening without wanting to judge you or fix you. Please let me know if there is anything I can do to help…" And then, in the quiet that follows, you can offer the genuine fondness of your heart to that region of your body. You don't need to force anything to happen, just relax and let your body be itself.

Now here is an interesting thing: it just so happens that the area deep inside your chest beneath your folded hands is a place that Wachiwi uses to communicate with us all the time…if we are listening. That area, called the solar plexus, has a whole vocabulary of sensations that can help us understand what Wachiwi needs and wants. We could even call it Wachiwi's "voice." And the more we pay attention to that area of our body, the more we will be able to understand what she desires to share with us. So after you become comfortable with the first exercise, you can expand it by consulting your solar plexus as you check in with various body regions. What sensations do you feel in your solar plexus in reference to your foot, hand, neck or back? What colors of light do you see when you look into your solar plexus with your eyes closed? What emotions do you feel? What images arise? Are there sounds or vibrations? Is there light? What does Wachiwi's voice have to say today?

There is another way of interacting with Wachiwi that can be helpful, and that is to imagine having a conversation with her in words. I will share with you how this has worked for me, just so you can get a feel for it. I have often imagined Wachiwi as a young girl of perhaps eight or nine strolling along beside me when I am going for a walk outside. At first, it seems important to just let her tag along in silence, without trying to start a conversation. Maybe I'll just look at her and smile. Or maybe I'll reach out my hand to see if she'd like to hold it while we walk. After a few minutes of companionable quiet, I will turn to her and say, "I'm glad you're here with me, Wachiwi." And I'll smile at her with my heart full of affection. If she frowns or looks away, I'll remain silent and just keep walking with her for a bit, then ask, "Wachiwi, is there something the matter? Would you like to tell me anything?" And then I will wait patiently to see if she says anything. If, on the other hand, she grins back at me, I will ask, "Wachiwi, how are you feeling? What would like to do today?" And then I will wait patiently for her to respond. Of course, she doesn't always respond right away. Sometimes it might not be until the very end of our walk – perhaps fifteen or twenty minutes later. But often she launches into how she is feeling right away, or starts babbling so hurriedly that I can barely keep up with her.

However we listen to Wachiwi, it is important to remember that we may not always understand what she is telling us. Even so, it is important not to interrupt her or make her feel that she has to explain herself all the time. If we don't understand, we can ask more questions, listen more attentively and openly, and try to feel our way through what she shares. Sometimes the most valuable aspect of our conversations with Wachiwi is just that we are paying attention to her and listening with an open heart. If we do understand what she tells us, then we should respond as compassionately and skillfully as possible. If she is hungry we should offer her food, sharing a meal with her; if she is tired we offer her rest and rest ourselves; if she wants to play then we can make time for her to play, and then join in the fun; if she wants to dance we let her dance, and we dance along; if she wants to hike up a mountain, we take her there and hike with her up its slopes.

Like any good parent, we can't always provide Wachiwi what she wants every time she asks. Sometimes we have to help her become more patient, explaining that yes, we can do what she wants later on, but not right now. Sometimes we might even have to be firm with her, and this may upset her. But part of being loving is sometimes saying "no." It also helps to have some structure in place to meet her most frequent requests. For example, if we always go for walks at certain times, eat at certain times, regularly sleep from this time to that time, and so on, then it will help Wachiwi feel reassured that her needs are indeed going to get met...even if we can't meet them right away. And because Wachiwi sometimes has a lot of needs, we may have to spread out the time we focus on her to different days of the week. But if she knows we will always eventually make time for her, she can be a more calm and content inner child. If we consistently follow through on our promises to her, she will know that she is loved and cared for. She will trust us.

Clear Intentions, Paying Attention, and Following Through

Before we meet some of our other inner children, I would like to explore some concepts that will help us become the best parents possible for all of them. These are meant to answer a central question, which is: "Why should I do these things at all?" What is really the point of caring for ourselves? Or creating balanced nourishment? Or listening to Wachiwi? What should our underlying motivations be for doing any of this...?

There are lots of reasons why I might want to improve how I care for myself. Maybe I am unhappy about some part of my life, and want to make things better. Maybe I recognize that parts of me want to heal and grow, but I'm not sure how to make that happen. Maybe I'm perfectly happy with the way things are, but I want to challenge myself further. In Integral Lifework, these are perfectly good reasons to get to know the different parts of self and explore ways of nourishing them. But Integral Lifework also encourages an additional motivation, called *the golden intention*.

The idea behind the golden intention is simple. Instead of focusing on what will benefit us as individuals, the golden intention encourages us to consider what will most benefit others, too. In fact, it urges us to consider that everything we think, say and do can have a positive influence on everyone and everything around us. It inspires us to pursue the greatest good for everyone as our primary motivation. This doesn't mean that we are only acting to benefit others, because we are part of that "All," so we will benefit as well. But focusing on "the good of All" shifts the main energy of our efforts away from self-centeredness, and into a more generous and compassionate spirit. Instead of asking ourselves "What is best for me right now?" we ask "What is best for everyone involved, both right now and keeping the future in mind?" or even "What is the wisest and most helpful thing I can do for the greatest number of people?" Ultimately, when we commit our thoughts, words and actions to the golden intention, we are asking the good of All to keep working through us.

How does this really work in practice, though? Well, let's look at nourishing Wachiwi as an example. Let's say I haven't been sleeping well, and Wachiwi has been very unhappy about this. As a result, I've become a little clumsy lately, bumping into things or even breaking things. I've been forgetting to do things that I promised others I would do. My thoughts have been fuzzy because I'm so tired all the time, and I haven't been able to listen very well to what others are trying to tell me. Because I am so sleep-deprived, I can't focus on doing my work, and I don't have much energy at the end of the day to do fun activities with my friends. Everything in my life is suffering...but everything my life touches is suffering, too. My friends feel like I'm not available for them. People who rely on me to get things done are beginning to wonder if their trust in me is deserved. Maybe I broke a loved one's favorite mug because of my clumsiness, or couldn't attend some event that was important to them because I was so tired. Maybe my absent-mindedness has injured others in ways I don't even know about. Perhaps because I was too tired to separate out the recycling from the garbage, or forgot to clean up some spilt paint before the rain washed it into the ground, I have even hurt the planet Earth in some way.

In this situation, if I have been measuring my own self-care through the lens of the golden intention – and encouraging Wachiwi to do the same – then my lack of sleep has hindered my ability to contribute to the good of All. I am not able to be the generous, attentive, loving person I want to be because I just don't have the energy or focus. So what motivates me to change this situation isn't just my own desire to care for myself, or my affection for Wachiwi, but also my desire to be a positive influence in the lives of others.

Now cultivating a guiding intention for the good of All does not, by itself, align our thoughts, words and actions with some sort of guaranteed outcome. It is just a beginning that helps inform our efforts. For our intentions to bear fruit, we also need to pay careful attention to how our thoughts, words and actions are fulfilling our intentions. In order to do this, I like to divide my "paying attention" into three specific times of day: when I first awake in the morning, in the present moment, and before I go to sleep at night. If I consciously summon the golden intention during those times, it will begin to imbed itself in my consciousness and persist throughout each day.

So in the morning, as I wake up, I will reflect on how I want to fulfill the golden intention over the course of the day. I will recall what I have committed to do for myself and others...for the good of All. For example, I might say, "I am going to go for a nice, long walk three times today, so that I am good and tired when I go to bed and can fall right to sleep. Whenever I go for a walk, I also become more alert and attentive because of the exercise, and this will help me be a better listener, and more productive in any work I do. Because I do this walking, I contribute more to the good of All." This is paying attention when I first awake. Over the course of the day, I will then revisit that commitment. "Have I gone for those long walks yet? No? Well, how about right now?" Then I will go for a walk, and while I am walking, I will reflect "This is fulfilling the commitment I made this morning." These are ways of paying attention to a commitment in the present moment. Then, at the end of the day, just before I go to sleep, I will reflect on how I fulfilled what I committed to do first thing in the morning, and why. "Did I go for three long walks? Was I more attentive to others because I exercised? Was I more alert? Was I more productive? Am I more tired now?" It is important that I avoid judging myself as I pay attention – I can always do better tomorrow regardless. This is simply about focusing my attention on my desired intentions and the reasons behind them.

And finally, all of this will have very little impact on my life if I lack the courage and discipline to follow through on what I intend. This courage and discipline can come from many different places. Ideally, it should result from the caring affection I feel for myself and others. But sometimes, if I just don't feel that affection in a given moment, I will need to rely on other things. Maybe I need to push myself by calling up a kind of stubborn resolve. "I'm going to do this!" I will say, and I will make myself follow through by force of will. Or maybe I will become irritated or even angry at myself for not following through, and I can use this to help me stick to the plan. Or maybe following through on something is making me feel nervous and afraid, so I will convince myself it doesn't matter, it's no big deal, I'll just do it without thinking about it and move on. Or maybe I'm just curious to see what will happen, and I'm willing to follow through to discover what awaits me on the other side! Sometimes, maybe I know from experience that, if I am persistent and keep trying, eventually it will become easier and easier to follow through. But regardless of where the courage and discipline come from – whether love, or curiosity, or anxiety, or detachment – I need to find a way to follow through...for the good of All.

Questions for Reflection & Discussion

- What kind of relationship do you feel you have with your Wachiwi right now? What are some of the reasons why you believe you have that relationship at this point in time?

- When was the last time you danced around for no particular reason? Or when was the last time you were able to be goofy, silly or carefree with your body? What would allow you to be that way? What might discourage you from being that way, and why?

- Can you look at your naked body in a mirror and feel okay with it, or do you feel there something you have to change? Why do you suppose you feel the way you do about your body?

- When you imagine Wachiwi within you, how many years old is she? Why do you think of her as being that age?

- Why is it sometimes important to withhold something your Wachiwi says she craves? How can we decide when it is best to encourage her natural appetites, and when it might not be?

- What are some reasons we might not always understand what Wachiwi is trying to tell us in a given moment?

- Do you feel your body is connected to Nature in any way? Do the rhythms of your body change with natural cycles of the sun, moon or seasons? How much time do you spend in Nature?

- What is the most nurturing thing you could do for your Wachiwi in the next twenty-four hours?

- Do you think having clear and consistent guiding intentions is important? Why or why not?

- What does "the good of All" mean to you? How would you describe it? What does it look and feel like?

Manjit the All-Knowing – Expanding the Mind

A name from India, "Manjit" (mahn-jeet) means *conqueror of the mind*. This sounds a little forceful or maybe even violent, doesn't it? And that's something we have to be careful about when we interact with Manjit, because he is in fact a conqueror, and often acts as if he wants our other inner children to follow his rules. Have you ever met someone who just loves to take control of every situation, telling everyone else what to do? Well, that's Manjit it a nutshell. And for most us, that's what Manjit actually gets to do a lot of the time. He'll even play elaborate tricks on us in order to have his own way. And while he's doing that, he will invent complicated reasons why he alone should always remain in control. Manjit can be a real handful!

At the same time, Manjit is just a kid like all our other inner children. He needs love, he needs to be nourished and encouraged, and he needs us to provide some discipline and structure to help him remain well. Also like our other inner kids, Manjit has some deeply ingrained habits he likes to follow, and various impulses or cravings over which he can obsess. Just like Wachiwi, Manjit wants to be active most of the time, constantly stimulated and constantly doing things. But instead of physical play, Manjit loves to think. He enjoys puzzles and questions without easy answers, and he can never get enough new information. For Manjit, knowledge isn't just facts about stuff, it's also how things are organized into categories, how each thing relates to other things, and how all of this fits together to make up a meaningful, sensible world. Whenever he encounters a geyser of knowledge spewing forth lots of information,

Manjit likes to run right in front of it, open his mouth, and try to swallow the whole blast as fast as he can.

As we discussed in the last chapter, if Wachiwi just ate junk food all of the time, she wouldn't be very healthy. In the same way, if we feed Manjit lots of fluffy, non-nutritional information, he'll gobble it up, but it won't be very healthy for him either. We could say that the difference between high quality information and fluff is the difference between education and just trying to escape into entertainment all the time. That is, to absorb real knowledge that is truly nourishing is different from filling our heads with exciting trivia. Of course, sometimes one person's trivia is another person's deeply held passion or life philosophy, so what defines valuable learning is going to be different from one person to the next. But it is important for us to separate one from the other for ourselves – according to what we value most – so that Manjit doesn't get lost in a desert of data that has no meaning or importance for our lives.

There is something else we must watch out for as well. Imagine a parent who told their child what to do all the time, without explaining why, and who threatened severe punishments if their child didn't obey them. You might hear them saying things like, "When I tell you to do something, just *do* it!" Or maybe "Don't question me, *just do as you're told!*" And because almost every household has some sort of routine, those harsh commands will tend to be repeated each and every day. "Put those dishes away!" Or "Time for bed. No questions." Or "Eat everything on your plate and don't talk back to me!" Or "Be quiet and go to your room!" Over time, repeating these kinds of commands over and over again turns them into something dangerous. They become patterns that are imprinted on a child's mind, making a young person respond reflexively and unquestioningly out of fear, performing the same tasks in endless repetition. Instead of learning to think for themselves, they become little robots controlled by anxiety and paranoia.

And just as it would be harmful to any child, these sorts of patterns are hurtful to Manjit. In order to thrive, he must be able to think for himself, explore for himself and find his way through new and exciting situations without always feeling anxious and afraid. This is what will make him strong and smart and inventive. If, as his parent, we take that freedom away from him, telling him he must *do this* or *think that* and not question our authority, it crushes his spirit. Also remember that, because Manjit likes to be in control, if we give him a rigid routine and tell him not to think, he will grab onto that routine because it gives him power. In other words, he will just turn around and use that routine to try to control our other inner children. For example, if we tell Manjit that red doolyhickuts are more valuable than blue doolyhickuts, and that he has to believe this or he will be punished, then he will go around telling everyone else that red doolyhickuts are the best. Red doolyhickuts rule. Red doolyhickuts are what life is all about. And everyone else better agree with him *or else*. Manjit will never even question whether such a thing as a doolyhickut exists…because he was never aloud to question.

So as his parent, it's our job to give Manjit the freedom and permission to ponder things, challenge us, and question what is true and real. We must encourage him to keep and open mind. What is a doolyhickut, after all? What is its function? Who invented doolyhickuts? Why are they important? Is there really any difference between red and blue doolyhickuts? Do doolyhickuts even exist…? We don't have to force Manjit to question things or keep and open mind – he will do this naturally, if we give him the space and time to do so, and reassure him that it's okay to be curious and open-minded. But if we notice that he is in a rut and repeating the same patterns over and over again, we may need to nudge him out of his rut into new territory. We may need to push him a little to look at things differently, to avoid having too much confidence in something he only half understands, and to try to appreciate each new idea from different points of view. All the while, we keep feeding him new information, introducing him to new comparisons between opinions and ideas, new insights into the world, new meanings and so forth. There is always more to learn, and there is an ever-growing world of ideas with new meanings and priorities.

Conversations with Manjit

Here is a curious thing about Manjit: because he really likes to be in control, sometimes he thinks *he* is the parent. He might even tell us we can just relax and let him handle everything. It is so easy for him to take over! So we have to be very careful not to let Manjit's enthusiasm override our better judgment. And one thing that will assist us in this is how we interact with Manjit each day, how we converse with him, and how we interpret his needs.

At first it may seem strange to think that one part of our mind can listen to another part of our mind, but this is actually a very valuable practice. We can think of it this way: Manjit is the portion of our mind that constantly absorbs new information, analyzes it, makes judgments about it, and then decides what to do in response. But there is another portion of our mind that can monitor Manjit from a distance, simply observing what he does from moment to moment. We could call this part of our mind "the Watcher." Have you ever seen a parent looking out a window as their child plays outside? That's the Watcher. Not involved, not trying to influence anything, just observing and considering.

If we aren't used to nudging our thinking in this direction, it can take some practice to get there. But once we've practiced for a little while, it becomes as easy as breathing. So, just as you did with Wachiwi in the previous chapter, take a moment to find a quiet place where you won't be disturbed, and sit with your eyes closed – or half-closed – looking inward without falling asleep. Remind yourself of the guiding intention that you are doing this "for the good of All." Sit comfortably with your hands resting lightly on your knees. Breathe deeply, evenly and slowly, and look inward into yourself. As thoughts, images and sensations naturally arise within your mind's eye, try to let them pass by without getting caught up in them. That is, without trying to figure out what they mean, or how you feel about them, or why they are there…just watching them arise. At first you might say to yourself, "Oh, look…there's a thought about what I'm going to have for lunch. And what's this? I'm worried about whether I'm doing this meditation correctly…isn't that interesting! Over here there seems to be a sort of itchy impulse to watch the movie I heard about last week…hmmm. And wow, I'm still upset about what my friend told me yesterday. Huh. What will I do about that tomorrow? Oh wait! That's me trying to distract myself from watching my thoughts without reacting to them! How funny…!"

Eventually, you will be able to let go of this inner dialogue, and just watch things unfold within your mind from a calm silence and without reacting at all. Again, this takes practice and persistence, but this is an invaluable tool for inner parenting. If we can remain uninvolved and just watch, we can learn what is really on Manjit's mind…what is interesting to him, what he is preoccupied with, what he yearns for and so on. We can also help him to slow down and relax a little – that is, help him let go of trying to monitor, analyze and control everything. At first Manjit may seem all-over-the-place, jumping from one memory, observation or idea to the next, but the more we remain calm, breathe deeply and evenly, and don't react to his flitting here and there, the more he can't help but slow himself down a bit. And once he has slowed down enough to be still, we can begin to have a meaningful conversation with him.

Now just as was true with Wachiwi, Manjit needs to know that we really care before he will confide in us. So while we are listening and watching, we should also remember to feel warmth and affection for Manjit – to really care about what he is thinking. Have you ever been speaking with someone and, in the midst of your conversation, had your mind start wandering somewhere else? Have you ever had someone ask, "So what do you think about that?" and been completely at a loss for how to respond, because you had accidentally stopped listening or become distracted by something else? Or have you ever had someone else space out while you were talking to them? This is what we want to avoid when interacting with Manjit, because as soon as he realizes our attention is somewhere else, we will lose his trust in that moment.

You might notice that there is a kind of contradiction happening here. On the one hand, I'm asking you to try to be aloof and distant from Manjit…watching him as if through a window without reacting to what he is doing. But on the other hand I'm asking you to engage him, to feel fond emotions for him, and demonstrate your caring with the quality of your attention. This is an important principle in parenting our inner children: we need to care enough to listen and assure them that they are loved, but we also need to remain distant and detached enough that we aren't caught up in their compulsions, frustrations and personal dramas. It is a balancing act of sorts, but if we allow ourselves to become overwhelmed by our inner children's experiences and reactions, we will not have the emotional strength or objectivity to help them choose a healthier course. We will not be able to love them skillfully.

As we try to walk this tightrope, we can begin asking Manjit about what is most important to him. We can't assume that whatever Manjit is obsessing over in any given moment is really important to him…Manjit might just be distracting himself. At some point we need to ask, "Manjit, what is really the most important to you? What do you really want right now? What can I help you with?" And then see what arises. Maybe Manjit will go right on processing what happened at the supermarket, or what he saw on TV, or dwell on something he learned recently that excited him, or maybe it won't be immediately clear what is the most important. But that's okay, just keep observing from a distance, breathing slowly and deeply, and feeling warm affection for Manjit. Wait for him to calm down and slow down, and ask again, "Is there anything you need that is more important than anything else…?" If you remain open and curious, without passing judgment on what Manjit has to offer you, he will eventually share what is dearest to him. This may take many attempts over many days, so patience and courage are your most reliable friends in this process. But over the course of many attempts, the mere fact that you are remaining so open and gentle with Manjit will nourish and encourage him, helping him feel safe and whole.

When Manjit does share what he wants, it then becomes your responsibility as a good parent to consider how healthy and productive his request really is. If all he wants to do is play games, we may need to encourage him gently in the direction of learning something new, like reading a book or watching a film that teaches him something he didn't know, or doing research about a topic he is unfamiliar with, or finding a solution to some problem. Even if he wants to do something that does enhance knowledge, if it is the same thing he always wants to do – or covers the same subject matter – perhaps we should mix it up a bit. Get him out of his comfort zone a little, and help him take a break from the same kinds of stimulation for a while. The more variation we can provide Manjit, and the more we can encourage him to remain open to new ideas and activities, the healthier and happier he will be.

We also need to directly address Manjit's desire to control everything and everyone else within us. For the less nourished he is, the more fiercely he will want to be in control. When he is trapped in the same inflexible routines, he will become more and more overconfident and arrogant, more and more eager to boss around the other children within.

And because this controlling impulse feels like power, Manjit will tend to reinforce his own ignorance – he will want to reject new information that challenges his previous understanding about things. For example, if he believes that there is breathable air in outer space, he won't want to accept that there isn't any air out there. If he thinks it's best to learn new information from watching reality TV, then he will resist learning from more accurate sources. So even though many of our inner children can be stubborn at times, Manjit is one of the most stubborn of all. Therefore, we have to be patient with him, and lead him gently and persistently to what is true and nurturing.

Now....did your mind wander at all when you read this chapter? Did you find yourself easily distracted by other things? Well, when we spend time observing Manjit in this way, two things can happen. The first is that Manjit becomes uncomfortable with the new direction you are taking him, and deliberately tries to disrupt the process. But that's okay, because as his parent you know what's best for him, and can gently steer him back to what is most important. Another thing that can happen is our other inner children may start clamoring for attention. For example, Wachiwi may say, "Can I talk to you right now? Can I? I have something I want to show you!" But this is Manjit's special time, and we need to remind our other inner children that they are all equally important, and will have their own special time, too. Just not right now. In this way we encourage mutual respect and appreciation between our inner children. By showing them that each deserves the same amount of love and care – the same special attention where we listen to their needs – we are demonstrating the harmony and balance necessary to achieve the good of All.

Questions for Reflection & Discussion

- Why do you think your Manjit wants to be so bossy and in control? What sort of tricks has Manjit played on you in the past so that he could continue telling you what to do?

- In terms of what you are feeding Manjit, what do you think the balance of entertaining fluff vs. high quality information is in your life? More fluff than high quality, or more high quality than fluff? Why do you think this is the case?

- Are there any set patterns that your Manjit likes to follow each day? Does he spend a lot of time thinking about the same sorts of things, even when he's supposed to be helping you with another subject or task? If either of these is true, why do you think that is?

- Why is it sometimes important to withhold something you're your Manjit that he craves? How can we decide when it is best to encourage his natural appetites and routines, and when it might be best to explore new territory?

- When you imagine Manjit within you, how many years old do you think he is right now? Why do you think that?

- What is one of your favorite mental activities, and how often have you been engaged in that activity during that past few weeks?

- For you, what is your Manjit most curious about? What questions does he want answered, and why?

- Do you remember your dreams when you wake up? Why or why not?

- What is the most nurturing thing you could do for Manjit in the next twenty-four hours?

ADELYTE THE ADORING – A HEART OF JOY

"Adelyte" (ah-deh-light) is a German girl's name that means *has good humor*. Adelyte is one of our inner children who feels things very deeply, and loves to express those feelings so everyone can share in them with her. She can't help herself – she is always bubbling over with emotion. When Adelyte feels loved and cared for, her heart soars with joy, and she shares that affection with everyone around her, especially her brothers and sisters. When she feels neglected or abused, Adelyte will cry out with hurt and despair, sometimes lashing out and even injuring herself or others. Her reactions can often be so intense that they drown out all our other inner children's voices and needs. But eventually, if we are a good parent to her, she will become more peaceful and content. And when Adelyte is happy, she can help keep all her brothers and sisters smiling, nurtured and entertained.

One of the most important things to realize about Adelyte is that, more than anything else, she wants to love and be loved. This is true with all our inner children to different degrees, but for Adelyte it is the air she breathes. If we nurture and sustain her, her loving affection and passionate devotion will continue to grow. How Adelyte expresses affection and passion will be unique for each person, but nearly always it will take some form of creative self-expression. Now I don't necessarily mean something artistic, like a perfect oil painting or a beautiful piece of music. She yearns to express herself, to connect with other people's hearts, and to be playful and free in how she does that. Whether she is yelling her innermost secrets at the top of her lungs, or whispering them softly, or shaping a silly-sounding poem around them, or baking a bright yellow cake that feels like the bright yellow joy within her, or tickling someone until they laugh in the same carefree way Adelyte herself is feeling, this girl needs to share her felt sense of the world with everyone – especially those closest to her. For Adelyte, every word and action is an opportunity to convey deepest feeling and invite others to experience those same emotions.

Of course Adelyte also wants to understand what is in other people's hearts as well. She wants to weave herself intimately into their lives, to feel what they feel, to walk in their shoes. If we let her, she will throw herself completely into someone else's situation just to appreciate their experience. Adelyte can be so curious and zealous that, if we don't help her set boundaries for those efforts – if we don't show her how to sometimes hold back and protect herself a little – she will become too caught up in other people's lives. So caught up that she can't remember who she is or how to function as an independent person. Adelyte will forget that, in order to love others fully, she must first become strong and secure in herself; she must be a separate, whole person who can love others without losing herself. So just as with all our other inner children, Adelyte has her own balancing act between two extremes: on the one hand shutting herself down and closing off her felt experiences, and on the other allowing the felt experiences of others to completely overwhelm or enslave her.

There is something else that excites and engages Adelyte, and that is being exposed to new emotions and experiences. Taking her for a trip to see new places can be thrilling for her. Or immersing her in some new activity, or meeting new people, or sharing new music, or experiencing performing arts she has never seen. Anything to remind her of all the different feelings available to her – excitement, apprehension, curiosity, shock, laughter, joy, sadness, wonder and so on. How about a ride at an amusement park? Or reading a story aloud to her? Perhaps meeting the neighbor's dog for the first time might do the trick. Of course, not everything that is new will be nourishing for Adelyte – some things may be too stressful or scary or overwhelming – but just the process of trying new things and exploring new emotions will help Adelyte grow and become stronger.

And, finally, for Adelyte there is nothing more sacred, precious and compelling than her relationships with others. Her relationship with you, her parent, is very important to her. As are her relationships with all her siblings, your other inner children. How you relate to others who are near and dear to you is essential to Adelyte's well-being. And Adelyte's relationships with ideas, principles and even moral values will become increasingly important to her as she gets older, too. Some of these relationships will be friendships, some of them will be love affairs, some of them will be relationships of convenience – like teaming up with an acquaintance to accomplish a short-term task – and some relationships may even become wide open, worshipful devotion. Adelyte can, should and will have many different types of relationships with every aspect of life. But what we need to realize as her parent is that her relationship with us is not necessarily the most important relationship she will have. This is sometimes hard to accept, because she is such an important and adorable member of our family, but sometimes Adelyte will be swept away with love for someone or something entirely foreign to us; sometimes she may even fall in love with everything and everyone at once. She will always love us as her parent, but she won't always keep us at the center of her universe, and we must allow her the freedom to find her own way in the world.

Conversations with Adelyte

Now here are some questions for you: How can you best nurture and sustain Adelyte? What can you do to assure her she is loved and cared for? How can you provide her with ways to express herself creatively and share her experiences with others? Are there ways you can help her have healthy, balanced relationships? And how can you encourage her to be open and carefree, without too many rules or burdens to weigh her down?

One place to begin is by practicing a special kind of inner attention. When Adelyte feels some emotions, it almost always surfaces somewhere in our physical body. Perhaps we feel stress as a tightness in the muscles of our neck. Or maybe joy is an upward rushing of warmth in the middle of our chest. When we are embarrassed, we might feel our face start glowing with heat. And when we are sad, we might sense our throat closing up, our chest becoming tight, and our eyes beginning to fill with tears. Isn't laughter a rush of air through our vocal cords? Isn't anger sometimes a clenching of fists and teeth? So if we pay careful attention to where our emotions are expressing themselves in our body, that is one very useful way of understanding what Adelyte is trying to tell us. And the more closely we listen, the more subtle those messages will be. For example, a very slight tensing of our stomach – something we might normally overlook – may inform us that Adelyte is worried or anxious about something. A subtle lifting sensation in our chest may remind us that Adelyte is excited about what is happening. Maybe a tiny sense of relaxation throughout our whole body will tell us that Adelyte is more content and at peace.

Another way to improve our connection and communication with Adelyte is by exposing her to different experiences, new people and varied forms of creative expression. Introduce her to some new tastes of food or drink. Take a class in some form of art or craft that you've always wanted to try, and see if Adelyte takes a liking to it. Bring her to a play or an art show. Share different kinds of music with her. Spend time with new people who have interests or aspirations that are similar to your own. In all of these situations, try to be as uninhibited as you can – that is, try to let go of any worries about what other people think and just be absorbed in the moment. Whether Adelyte is active or passive in these situations, they provide her an opportunity to set herself free, to share what she feels and longs for, and to experience what other people feel and long for.

Another way we can connect with Adelyte is to encourage her to refine her emotional vocabulary. This will help Adelyte express herself to you and to others more easily and accurately. It will also help her understand and empathize with the emotions of others. For example, what is the difference between frustration and anger? Or between contentment and elation? Or between grief and sadness? How can we tell the difference between a grimace of distaste and a grimace of physical effort on someone else's face? Or between a shrug that means "I give up" verses a shrug that means "I don't know"? How can we tell the difference between a genuine smile and a false or saccharin smile? As you learn about various shades of emotion, you can invite Adelyte to recognize them in herself and others. Then, when she needs to express a specific emotion, or appreciate what someone else is going through, she will have a larger vocabulary to work with.

Adelyte may communicate with us in many different ways. The most important for us is being ready to listen, and to respond with openness and a willingness to act. If Adelyte wants to cry, we should allow the tears to flow. If Adelyte is angry about something, we should find healthy ways to express that anger. If Adelyte is bursting with joy, we should find ways to set that joy free into the world. If Adelyte longs to sing or write or draw pictures, we should sing or write or draw with her. At some point, we may also want to explore why she is feeling a certain way, perhaps even starting a dialogue with her, but allowing those emotions to spill out of us is one of the most caring and compassionate things we can do for this inner child. Are there times when we will want to contain the intensity of Adelyte's reactions, or delay their expression until a later time? In certain social situations this may be the case, and a part of helping Adelyte grow and mature is learning how to delay or moderate strong reactions that may not be helpful in-the-moment. But, eventually, we will always need to find a way to allow Adelyte share herself with others, no matter what kind emotion she is feeling.

Just as with all our children, we provide Adelyte the Adoring with both freedom and structure. The freedom to be herself, and the structure to be herself in the most constructive and nourishing ways. The freedom to feel deeply and powerfully, and the structure to channel those feelings into helpful and supportive expression. For example, if Adelyte is furious about something, you can take her for a long walk or run or bike ride, and that anger can fuel your muscles until they get tired and the anger calms. If Adelyte is excited about some new idea, you can write about it or share that excitement with a friend. If Adelyte is fiercely in love with someone, you can find ways to express that love while not overwhelming the object of her affections. I also try to avoid telling Adelyte that she's not supposed to feel a certain way – she feels what she feels! And whatever form of expression that emotion takes is completely up to us. As her parent, it is simply your responsibility to help Adelyte express herself in ways that enrich everyone and harm no one. With the golden intention as your guide, the universe of emotions within can add precious energy to the good of All.

Questions for Reflection & Discussion

- Do you feel that your Adelyte is loved as much as she would like to be? Why or why not?

- Do you feel that your Adelyte is full of love for others? Why or why not? Has she been able to express that love regularly?

- Does your Adelyte have enough freedom to fully be herself and express all aspects of herself – all her various many of emotion? Why or why not?

- What about structure? Do you believe your Adelyte has enough structure to feel safe and self-disciplined when she needs to be?

- Are there ever times when you might want to discourage Adelyte from feeling a certain feeling, at least for a little while?

- What is one of your favorite heart-centered activities, and how often have you been engaged in that during that past few weeks?

- For you, what does Adelyte most long for? What is most important to her, and why?

- How would you rate the quality of your Adelyte's relationship with others? Does she feel connected? Why or why not?

- Has Adelyte ever become so involved in some passionate interest, or in the concerns of someone else, that she has forgotten to care for herself? If so, why do you think this has happened?

- What is the most nurturing thing you could do for your Adelyte in the next twenty-four hours?

SHEN OF THE SPIRIT – TOUCHING OUR INNER LIGHT

When used as a boy's first name, the Chinese "Shen" (shen) means *spiritual, deep thinking.* As a term in Chinese religious studies, "shen" has the broader meanings of *spirit, deity, spiritual, supernatural, awareness,* and *consciousness.* In all these senses, Shen is the perfect name for the child within that lives, breathes and perceives the spiritual realm. Unlike some of our other inner kids, Shen does not always make his presence known to us. He can often be found in quiet corners just out of sight, alternately watching his brothers and sisters with affectionate intensity, then drifting off into a sort of daydream where he barely seems present at all. He can be a very difficult child to get to know, mainly because he sees things so differently than our other children. He is wise beyond his years, but often keeps quiet about what he knows. And since many of his habits are inexplicable or mysterious to us at first, it can take a while to develop a strong bond of trust with him.

What does Shen yearn for? He yearns for a very special kind of connection: a personal connection with what is sometimes called "our spiritual ground of being." What is this spiritual ground he wants to connect with? Well, it has different names and descriptions among different languages and cultures around the world. Some describe it as *soul* – our individual soul, or a part of the great soul of the Universe itself. Others describe it as a mysterious force behind all things, creating and energizing all life. Still other traditions define spiritual ground as the essence or fundamental substance of everything that exists. Others relate to spiritual ground as our connection with the Divine, a communion with Deity that is always available inside us. And other belief systems view the ground of being as the potential for spiritual liberation – the seed of enlightenment – that exists within all beings. I myself consider this spiritual ground a sort of bridge, a conduit of spiritual energy and knowledge, which channels the energies and insights from the invisible realm of spirit into the visible world of matter. A bridge of Light that connects the mysterious impulse that sets the Universe in motion with the ordinary motions of our daily lives. But however we define it, what Shen desires most is to spend quality time interacting with that bridge to mystery; he longs to feel that inner Light warming his face and heart.

Perhaps you already have learned to relate to your inner Light in some specific way. For example, perhaps you have learned some form of prayer or meditation. And that's great! Now here's a precious secret about the life of Shen: he is actually connected to our spiritual ground of being all the time, but we often aren't paying careful attention to what he's doing. Just like Wachiwi is always on the verge of dancing, and Manjit is always processing and evaluating, and Adelyte is always feeling her way through things, whether we realize it or not Shen is having some sort of spiritual conversation and connection with the Universe nearly all of the time. As Shen's parent, our main concern then becomes the quality and intensity of that conversation and connection, and our willingness to participate in the process. We want to encourage him to delve deeper, understand more completely, and experience more fully. For just like our other children, if Shen is ignored, neglected or otherwise made to feel unimportant, he can become confused and hurt, and end up not receiving all the nourishment he needs to thrive. So as Shen's parent, it is our responsibility to provide him a little compassionate guidance and structure.

Another important aspect of parenting Shen is encouraging him to express his spiritual experiences in concrete actions. Many spiritual experiences can be very positive and uplifting, inspiring us toward greater compassion and caring for ourselves and others. For even if we were to live inside a blissful bubble of spiritual Light all the time, that experience will not be helpful or meaningful unless we translate it into action. Inner bliss must be channeled into outer blessings. One of the easiest ways to do this is to practice generosity and service – to give our time, energy and resources to those in need. Shen already wants to do this, but he is understandably nervous. Perhaps he fears rejection a little, or is unsure about being skillful or wise enough to serve others in effective ways. If we can take those first steps to become a blessing presence to others, we will be able to help Shen overcome his fear and celebrate his vibrant spirit.

Conversations with Shen

We can start our conversations with Shen by creating the same conditions we did in the previous chapters for our other children. We begin by finding quiet place to sit uninterrupted; breathing deeply and evenly with our eyes closed; focusing our attention inward; and encouraging stillness. And, as we have in those other parenting efforts, our main role is to be an encourager and nurturer, full of love and affection, while at the same time learning to letting go. That is, not forcing Shen to do one thing or another, but gently and patiently nudging him toward our inner Light. There are a number of ways we can do this – so many in fact that hundreds of books have been written about different spiritual practices – but I believe all of them ultimately lead to the same place. The following exercise combines a handful of these different practices into one method, and builds on the practices you worked on in previous chapters. With patience and the courage to persist, it can help you strengthen the Shen within you.

Now before we explore this practice, I want to revisit an important idea: having a "guiding intention" in everything we do; a state of mind and heart that you create within yourself as you engage the practice. When someone who really loves to play a sport is about to begin playing, they are often full of excitement and an inner commitment to do their very best. When a passionate musician is about to play or sing or compose, their heart is likewise filled with a desire to express the beauty and perfection of the music and its emotional meaning. When I stand before a class of students, I want to communicate the full and complete body of thought in my mind – I want them to understand me and not be confused. These are examples of having a guiding intention. As we discussed in the chapter on Wachiwi, the guiding intention I would like to promote here is both simple and profound. It is a desire that the outcome of all the practices in this book be positive and beneficial for everyone and everything; the golden intention.

This desire for the good of All is mainly about feeling a strong sense of compassion and goodwill towards everyone and everything. When we really care about a pet, we don't want it to get hurt or to suffer in any way – we want it to thoroughly enjoy its existence. When we really care about another person, we likewise want what is best for them. When we really care about the Earth, we don't want to destroy or pollute it, but maintain an inner intention that the entire Earth will live, grow and flourish. When we really care about ourselves, we are committed to self-nurturing so that we can be happy, peaceful and successful in life. A desire for the good of All combines all of these kinds of caring intentions. So whenever we begin our conversations with Shen, those conversations will be much more powerful and effective if we hold this golden intention in the forefront of our heart and mind.

Here is one meditative practice we can use to connect with our spiritual ground of being, fully nourishing our Shen:

Once you have found a quiet place to sit and relax, begin your meditation with an inner commitment to the golden intention, i.e. "May this be for the good of All." It will be helpful to be in the same place, and seated in the same position, each time you begin this practice. Being in the same place and position helps all our inner kids realize that it is time to pursue a specific outcome or process.

Relax every part of your body. Start with your hands and feet – perhaps moving them or shaking them a little to release tension – then your arms and legs, then your torso, head and neck.

Breathe deeply and evenly deep into your stomach, preferably in through the nose and out through the mouth, so that your shoulders remain still but your stomach inflates. Purse your lips slightly and allow your cheeks to puff up as you exhale. Practice this until you are comfortable with it in a steady rhythm.

With your mind's eye centered in the very middle of your chest, between your backbone and the bottom of your ribs, silently ask

yourself **"Where is now?"** Don't worry about exactly what this means for now, just ask the question with an open mind. Slowly search within yourself for a physical location for the present moment. As words, images, feelings or experiences arise within you, create lots of room for them in your mind and heart without trying to decide what they mean – just sit with them for a moment and then let them go. Remember to breathe deeply and evenly. Always return to the question "Where is now?" and, rather than expecting a clear or rational answer, be open to feelings and sensations, which hint at answers that are deeper than thought. The goal here is to delve beneath surface experiences, to brush against something at the very depths of our being.

If you practice for fifteen minutes and nothing seems to be happening, just relax and keep going. As with other nourishing practices, sometimes it is easy to become distracted or bored, but just keep breathing and questioning, perhaps changing how you ask the question. For example, try shifting the emphasis on each word, such as: *"Where* is now?" or "Where *is* now?" or "Where is *now?"* Repeat each new emphasis several times. Remember to keep the good of All as your primary intention, and don't worry about any sort of special or momentous result occurring. Just try this new approach for as long as you can, and see what happens.

Remember that touching your inner Light is a different experience for everyone. For some people strong emotions may be involved. For others a different way of thinking or perceiving may occur. Some people experience physical sensations. And other people observe a fading away of all sensations and awareness, as if certain parts of the mind and body are falling asleep. If you don't sense anything happening, even after several attempts on different days, you can always try one of the many techniques offered by different spiritual traditions. For example, something else you can experiment with is to pause in your breathing – at the end of both each inhale and exhale – for about the length of a breath. This isn't supposed to be a forced or uncomfortable sort of rhythm, but a relaxed way to coax your breathing into four parts – a "four-fold" breath of in, rest, out, rest. It may take some practice to remember the words, the guiding intention, and the breathing all at once...but keep at it until you find a comfortable balance. If you do decide to try a different spiritual practice, remember that it is helpful to wait a day or two before trying anything new.

As thoughts, feelings, sensations or images arise during your practice, just relax into them for a few moments, and then let them go. What I mean by "let them go" is to release any interest you might have about what is going on inside you, and open your mind and heart so each event can just fly away. You might resist wanting to let go of certain things, and that's okay, but keep trying to relax your grip on whatever you may be holding onto. One thing that can help is to breathe out whatever image, thought or feeling seems to be sticking inside. You could also encourage other inner sensations – bright light, loud pleasing sounds, or strong emotions – to overwhelm whatever is stuck in your meditative attention. Remember to avoid being to forceful or fearful in rejecting what happens inside you – be careful not to deny or repress what you encounter. Just allow your interior to be spacious, receptive and open to whatever comes. Be comfortable in not knowing what will happen, and gradually let go of your anxiety and fear.

If, even after a half hour or more of four-fold breathing or alternate phrasing, your mind still drifts away from interior spaciousness and stillness, trying switching to "Where is now?" as a mantra. That is, repeat it evenly, several times with each breath, either aloud or silently. As in "whereisnowwhereisnowwhereisnow...." over and over again. Remain focused on the rhythm of the words rather than their meaning. Maintain an even, slow, relaxed rhythm of breathing – or the four-fold breath if you can do that. And remember to hold the golden intention gently in your heart. Once again, as you repeat the mantra, acknowledge whatever arises without passing judgment on it, and then let it go.

At some point, after a number of practice sessions where you have trained yourself to follow these steps without resistance, you will experience a sense of arriving at a new place. Different people describe this arrival in different ways, with different sensations and levels of intensity. It also tends to require different amounts of practice time for different people. However, you will recognize on some level that you have encountered "right now" in a new form. In fact, this arrival can occur so suddenly that it jolts you out of your breathing and focus. If this happens, just relax and return to the rhythm of words and breath, and to the spaciousness and stillness within yourself. Immerse yourself in this place for as long as possible, always remembering to breath in and breath out. Know that you are safe, and continue to let go.

There are lots of things that can derail this practice. For example, if any particular thing keeps resurfacing during your inner focus over and over again (a concept, an image, and emotion, a sensation, etc.), and you just can't seem to let it go, take a break. Instead, try confronting the resurfacing experience directly. Challenge it with questions: "What are you? Where are you coming from? What do you want? Why are you here?" And so on. Allow some openness in yourself for a response, and rest in that response just as you sat with other sensations that arose within. Then, whatever answers come, let those go as well. Always remember to breathe. If you become really upset, physically uncomfortable, jittery, dizzy or disoriented, relax through those situations as best you can. However, if uncomfortable sensations or experiences persist or become extreme, stop all practice for the day, and try again in a day or two.

No matter what happens during this practice, always give yourself time and space after your meditation to process what you have experienced. Open your eyes and just *be* with what has happened without judgment or a sense of coming to definite conclusions for several minutes. This is where Shen can help us process what we have experienced, where we can give thanks for his participation, where we can sit quietly by his side, embracing him with warm affection. Like any child, when we open ourselves to Shen's curiosity and insights, we will learn from him. As any parent will tell you, paying careful attention to what children share with us allows them to become our teacher; as we care for them, they in turn care for us in ways we never could have expected. Encouraging our inner children to explore their particular strengths, gradually learning how to best nourish themselves, is what will keep us centered, anchored, and always moving forward.

You might be wondering why I am offering so many careful specifics in this exercise, especially as contrasted with previous chapters, and there is an important reason for this. It is mainly because the modern world has become very good at distracting us from this kind of inner attention, and it often takes serious and disciplined effort to help us rediscover it. It is much easier to pick up a book, or listen to a podcast or radio broadcast, or watch a video, or interact with folks online, or play a game, or hang out with friends. It is much easier to engage in habitual patterns of work, carefree activities, or passionate obsessions than it is to shine a bright light on our inner world. These other activities can nourish our inner children in different ways, but they may also make it easier to avoid the nourishment Shen requires.

Finally, remember that the second part of this process is to translate whatever you have experienced in your conversations with Shen into action. For example, if your meditation helps you feel warm and affectionate, then express that warmth and affection towards someone soon after you finish. If you feel more calm and centered, then demonstrate that through increased patience and understanding for other people. If you have an "aha" moment, where you realize something meaningful for your life, share that *aha* with a friend. If you experience an increased sense of kindness and caring in your practice, then demonstrate it with generosity towards others. And so on. Whatever you experience, find ways to share it with the world.

Questions for Reflection & Discussion

- What has your relationship with Shen been like? Have you experienced a regular connection with your spiritual ground of being?

- Why do you think it might be important to translate spiritual experiences into action? Why could it be helpful to express spiritual bliss as a blessing presence to others?

- Do you think service and generosity are healthy ways to express a connection with your inner Light? Why or why not? If so, how do you envision yourself becoming a "blessing presence" to others?

- Do you think having an underlying, guiding intention is important to your spiritual practice? Why or why not?

- What is one of your favorite spiritual activities, and how often have you been engaged in that during that past few weeks?

- When and why do you think it would be appropriate to take a break from any sort of conscious spiritual practice?

- Do you think the modern world distracts us from our relationship with Shen? Why or why not?

- Do you think all types of spiritual practice lead us to the same place? Why or why not?

- What is the most nurturing thing you could do for your Shen in the next twenty-four hours?

LIVELY LUCERIA – LEARNING TO BE FLEXIBLE

"Luceria" (loo-sehr-ee-ah) is a Latin name that means *circle of light*. Luceria is a wonderfully caring and attentive inner child, who is intensely interested in making sure that there is harmony and peace in the family. She is like a dutiful older sister who wants to help with the parenting of her younger siblings, but is so concerned with this that she often ends up trying to please everyone, helping them all feel happy and content, while forgetting to care for herself. Also, because she so wants to please, what often happens is that Luceria's efforts are ruled by whatever inner child is strongest in-the-moment. For example, if one of our other inner children tends to be our favorite, or we are constantly preoccupied with parenting one child because they are so demanding, Luceria will focus all of her attention wherever we are focusing all of our attention. As a result, Luceria herself can work so hard to please our neediest child that she all but forgets about the other members of our inner family. Very quickly, all the relationships in the household can become so out-of-balance that nothing seems to be running smoothly anymore. Often, the result is that no one is happy.

However, because Luceria is such a good helper, all we need to do to set things right is remind her of the importance of the balance and flexibility she also prizes. If we set clear priorities for who gets nourished when, Luceria will become an invaluable support in making that happen. Also, because she is so talented at enabling harmony in our being, she can in turn remind us of when we are focusing too much attention on one child and neglecting others – that is, *if we remember to listen to her*. So, as with all of our other inner relationships, it is important for us to trust her insight as well as demonstrate to her that we are a trustworthy and caring parent.

In addition to helping maintain balance and equal attention within our family, Luceria also has another unique gift: she can help us shift effortlessly from one primary mode of interaction to another. What do I mean by "mode of interaction?" Well, so far we have explored how our body (Wachiwi), heart (Adelyte), mind (Manjit) and spirit (Shen) can best be nourished. As we nurture each of these children, we are effectively switching from one primary mode of interaction to another mode. For example, when we are interacting with Wachiwi, we are in a physical mode. Then we interact with Manjit in a mental mode. We interact with Adelyte in an emotional mode, and with Shen in a spiritual mode. Each is like a unique language that each child understands better than any other, and as their parent we must learn to speak all of them fluently.

These different modes of interaction are really different ways of being, and rely on different parts of our consciousness to process what is happening. In this sense, you could think of "consciousness" as the total of all your parts of self that perceive, bring together, express and remember everything that is happening around you. One way to understand this is that you see with your eyes, hear with your ears, feel with your skin and smell with your nose, but you take in whatever happens around you with all of these senses at once, and without really thinking about your individual senses. It is the total of all of our senses that allows us to perceive some event in all its completeness. Have you ever been outside in a thunderstorm? There is a flash of lightening, the damp patter of rain on the skin, the fresh smell of rain-wet earth, and the resounding crack of thunder. But none of these things by itself conveys the completeness of the storm. All of them combine into what we sense and understand to be *a thunderstorm*.

But here's the catch: often we tend to depend on one of our senses more than another. We might rely more on sight than hearing, or more on touch than smell, and so on. This is natural, especially in certain situations. If some surface feels like it is very hot, it doesn't matter if there is no burning smell or glow of heat, we will avoid resting our hand on that surface to avoid injury. If some food we are about to eat smells like it is spoiled, it won't matter if it looks okay, or feels normal to the touch, because the smell alone tells us that eating it could be hazardous. If we see two people we know talking to each other across the street, we may not be able to hear the sound of their voices or smell their unique scents, but we recognize them and wave to them anyway. Learning to rely on different senses to make decisions in different situations is an important skill.

In the same way, learning to rely on different modes of interaction in different situations is also important; we can't always rely on one mode to understand or accomplish everything. Unfortunately, the modern world has a tendency to force us into one primary mode of interaction most of the time, and so other modes can become rusty, slow or neglected altogether. For instance, at school or work I might be asked to do lots of mental calculating and quick decision-making to navigate each task, to figure out everything that is going on around me using a mainly mental mode of interaction, while relying on little else. In my relationships with my family, it may seem like all of my decisions are expected to come from an emotional mode of interaction, with very little input from the logical part of my brain, my spiritual insights or my physical intuition. Whenever I talk to friends about my romantic interests, they may encourage me to make romantic decisions solely on my physical or emotional attractions. And so on. In each case, other modes of interaction are made to seem less important.

And of course Luceria learns how to relate to the world and our other inner children through many of these day to day interactions. Perhaps she also sees how people interact on a TV show, or in a book, and tries to imitate that. She may also hear advertisements that claim a perfume fragrance can enhance romance. She may see people all around her trying very hard to look and act a certain way, and hear them being critical of others who aren't trying to look and act that way. In the workplace, she may observe that people with the most power seem very cold and intellectual in their decision-making, and who are uncaring or dismissive of people who operate in different modes of being. But all of these ways of interacting are one-dimensional – they incorrectly assume that only certain modes of interaction – emphasizing heart, or mind, or body or spirit as the preferred primary mode – are more appreciated and expected in particular circumstances. This is one of the most unfortunate lies of the modern culture, because we really should be connecting with other people and our environment with our whole self. All of our inner kids should be allowed to participate at any time.

For in order for Luceria to flourish, she must be allowed to move effortlessly through all modes of interaction, to combine them in different ways when needed, and to be fluid and flexible in any situation. No mode of interaction should be considered superior to any other – they are all equally important, just as all our inner children are equally important. Whenever we tell her "You need to operate this way in this situation, and that way in this other situation, without any flexibility!" we are turning Luceria into a sad, stiff, limited little robot. We are crushing her spirit. So instead, we must encourage her to explore all modes of interaction in all situations, and not feel pressured or rushed by others to confine herself to just one or two. We must place all of our inner resources at her disposal. But how can we do this?

Conversations with Luceria

If we can provide Luceria with the space and time to find her own way, she will make good decisions. She will show us how we can best support and nourish her. Part of this means that we will let go of old habits or avoid environments, interactions and activities that take away her freedom to choose – especially if they take it away for long periods of time. I might be a very gifted chess player, but if all I ever do is play chess, I will not be a very complete human being. I might enjoy interacting with people socially, but if that is all I ever do, then other parts of me will never develop. I might be a fast runner, but if all I ever did was run as fast as I can, I would never really get anywhere in this life. So sometimes, to provide Luceria with space and time, all we need to do is stop taking it away from her – by setting aside for a little while anything that demands a constant and singular focus.

Along these lines, two of the strongest allies to help us hear and empower Luceria are the practices of *resting* and *fasting*. Resting means just that: taking time out, stopping whatever we are doing for a few minutes, breaking from our focus or shifting our routine. And this doesn't just mean physical rest, but mental rest, emotional rest, spiritual rest, social rest, resting from our purpose, and so on. In other words, resting in every dimension of our being. Sometimes this happens in a sort of trade-off between one inner child and another. I might rest my mind by going for a walk, or rest my body and mind by sleeping, or rest my social interaction with alone time, and so on. Sometimes, though, resting isn't enough, because it doesn't provide the amount of space and time Luceria needs to fully shift our mode of being. Sometimes we need to fast. Fasting is a simple process that extends and amplifies the idea of resting. But instead of just switching our mode for a few minutes or hours, we switch it for a few days. We avoid strenuous physical effort for a week or more. We avoid our favorite entertainment for a month. We spend several days alone in the wilderness without any contact with other people. We stop engaging in intense arguments or intellectual debates for a few months. We let go of our regular nourishment routine and mix things up, providing lots of peaceful, quiet space for Luceria to work her magick. Using these two tools – resting and fasting – we can create strong and lasting harmonies, even if we are feeling chaotic, compulsive or far out-of-balance.

Another practice that helps Luceria is to engage in activities that are carefully unstructured, but that stimulate different modes of interaction at the same time. Taking a long walk alone in Nature, or just sitting for a while out in the wilderness, or paddling a boat on open water for a few hours...all of these are ways we can allow Luceria to take over and encourage balance. The key is not having any agenda, not having a specific destination or goal, and spending that unstructured time apart from other people (or at least not interacting with anyone!). Spending time alone, without any specific activity that demands a certain kind of attention, allows us to hear Luceria's voice if we are open to it. Then again, if we spend all of that unstructured time thinking about our schedule tomorrow, or what we are going to say to a loved one when we return home, or how we are going to finish our latest creative project, this will keep us distracted from listening for her voice.

The final contributor to Luceria's balancing process is becoming fully present to what is happening right here, right now. Sometimes, if we are used to operating in a particular mode, we will slip right back into that mode even as we try to escape it. This is why making sure we are spending time with each of our inner children is so important: those interactions teach us how to switch modes. When we play with Wachiwi, we learn how to communicate with our bodies. When we express our creativity with Adelyte, we get in touch with the heart's modes of being. When we stimulate our mind with learning, Manjit shows us how to process things in our head. And when we embrace our ground of being, Shen shows us what spiritual processing looks and feels like. Then, when we spend time alone in Nature or unstructured activities, we can recognize whatever modes we happen to be operating in, encouraging and supporting each one. When we do this, it is like taking a vacation and allowing everyone time to rest. And the quality of that rest is such that Luceria has time to nourish herself, instead of feeding everyone else.

If this type of "inner vacation" seems challenging for you, there are also some structured approaches that may help. Most of them involve some sort of body-centered practice to achieve a restful, neutral state. Examples of widely available techniques include things like Tai Chi, Hatha Yoga and Qigong. Really, though, anything that helps us focus on the now – including the different practices found in this book – can be beneficial. And once we learn to allow Luceria freedom in how she balances the flow and frequency of our interactions within and without, she will in turn nourish, strengthen and support all other dimensions of self. As one sample practice, you could try the following "wandering" exercise.

As with all such exercises, it is helpful to set your intention before you begin by feeling and saying, "May this be for the good of All." Then, to free up your modes of interaction, take a walk in an environment that is unfamiliar to you, without a clear destination or time limit. Make sure that it is a safe environment – and that you can contact help if you become lost! Begin by deciding which way to go – left, right or straight – without a logical or a deliberate objective. Instead, try to feel your way through each change in direction, noting the sensations deep in the middle of your chest and the pit of your stomach as you consider which direction to go. Do you feel a lifting, freeing sensation for one direction? Try going that way. Do you feel a clenching sensation? Try avoiding that direction. See what happens. At some point you may lose your sense of place and time altogether as you follow your inner promptings –

and that's great! It means you are becoming absorbed in the now, and providing Luceria with the rest, spaciousness and neutrality she needs to create balance. Now, once you have become fully absorbed in the present moment, how long can you remain there...?

Questions for Reflection & Discussion

- What has your relationship with Luceria been like? Have you been able to maintain a balance of attention and effort among all your inner children?

- Can you recognize when you shift from one primary mode of interaction to another? For example, from a mental mode to an emotional mode, or a spiritual mode to a mental mode?

- Are you aware of certain social situations or environments where you are expected to rely mainly on just one or two modes of interaction? Are there certain events, relationships or places where you feel like you are expected to "turn off" certain modes of being altogether?

- What types of unstructured activities do you think will encourage inner balance, stimulate multiple modes of interaction, or inspire your Luceria to express her needs more fully?

- What modes of interaction are easiest or most familiar for you? What are the most difficult? Why do you think one mode is easier, and another more difficult?

- Why might it be beneficial to train ourselves away from relying on a mode of being that is most familiar or comfortable to us?

- Can you describe what it feels like to shift from one mode of interaction to another? What sensations or emotions are present? In contrast, what does it feel like to enter a neutral or resting space, where any or all modes could be engaged if you wanted, but none currently are?

- What is the most nurturing thing you could do for your Luceria in the next twenty-four hours?

ENTANGLED EILON – CREATING A SUPPORTIVE COMMUNITY

"Eilon" (eye-lawn) is a Hebrew name that means *oak tree*. Eilon is a very socially active child; he longs for interaction and connection with others on every level. To laugh and play, to talk and listen, to hold hands or wrestle, to agree or debate, to go on an exciting adventure or seek quiet comfort – everything is worthwhile for Eilon if it includes other people. In all of this he wants to help others succeed, and hopes that others will help him too. He especially enjoys seeing other people support and encourage each other for no other reason than to celebrate each others' joy. For Eilon, a perfect world is one in which everyone he cares about always feels connected and actively engaged with each other. It's not enough for Eilon to take pleasure in something alone, he just has to share it. Whether it's a great book, some delicious food or a funny joke, Eilon lives to see others benefit from sharing in the experience. What nourishes Eilon to his very core is a feeling of belonging, of constant giving and receiving within a larger group.

What gets Eilon in trouble sometimes, however, is that he isn't always wise and discerning about which groups to join, or who to make friends with, or when to share his most personal secrets. Because his yearning for connection is so strong, sometimes that yearning overwhelms his better judgment. This can lead to unfortunate outcomes, where Eilon gets hurt by his experiences with other people – sometimes so much so that he wants to withdraw from any kind of relationship at all. So our role as his parent is to guide him into safe and productive interactions with others, to help him develop healthy social boundaries and understand how to navigate them, and to protect him from becoming so invested in friendship, romantic or community commitments that he loses himself, becomes overwhelmed, or doesn't allow other inner kids to be nourished. Given the opportunity, Eilon will inevitably entangle himself in his relationships – that is predictable. But we can assist him by being more skillful in how we interweave his life with the lives of others, so that his experience will always be nurturing and enriching.

One way we can support Eilon's efforts to connect with others is to educate ourselves about codependence, and how to overcome it. What is codependence? It is a set of behaviors and responses that may appear kind or caring on the surface, but are actually quite harmful. They are harmful because they are rooted in a set of mistaken beliefs about what caring and kindness are supposed to look and feel like.   For example, perhaps I believe that tightly controlling someone else's behavior will protect them from harm. And because I am protecting them this way, I call it "love." But really I am enslaving them to my own fears and worries. A more compassionate way of interacting would be to provide someone I love with information about the risks and benefits of a given situation, a few options I think might be skillful or successful, and then let them decide for themselves what to do. This way, instead of taking away their freedom and power of choice, I help them appreciate the most constructive ways to use that freedom and power, and then let go.

Another way codependence can show up is when our own emotional state or well-being is tied too closely with someone else's. If we can only feel happy when someone else is happy, or always become angry or distraught when someone we care about is angry or distraught, or can't be satisfied or at peace if someone else has even the slightest discomfort, these indicate a codependent pattern. We might also believe it is our responsibility to make sure other people are okay and fix all of their problems for them, always making sure we've done our part before we allow ourselves to relax. Often this leads to a strong desire to avoid all conflict or uncomfortable emotions, and leads us to assume that being nice is the same as being kind. This type of codependent says, "if I can change my own behavior to ensure there is peace and tranquility, then that is what I must do, and I am not allowed to ask for anything in return."

So codependence is really all about either trying to control other people, or allowing ourselves to be controlled by other people, usually in order to feel tranquil, safe or empowered. Overcoming codependence may require healing on many levels. However, one solution is to consistently aim for authentic empathy and compassion, and let go of any desire to control or be controlled.   After that, if we continue to assess the outcomes of our efforts, we will know how authentic our kindness really is.   This requires a change in our fundamental beliefs about where happiness and contentment come from. For in reality they do not come from relationships with other people, but from how we relate to ourselves. Happiness and contentment are grounded in the compassion and affection we feel for all our inner children, and for the total self that is greater than the sum of its parts. Eilon may not want to accept this at first, because his focus is all about connecting with others; for him the intoxication of social connection feels like the key to joy and lasting satisfaction. But this is an illusion, and the sooner we begin to nourish Eilon and all of our inner kids in loving harmony, the sooner we will experience more authentic empathy and compassion towards others.

We've already touched upon some aspects of authentic compassion in previous chapters, because the most effective ways to care for our inner children are founded on real loving kindness. True compassion is being accepting and tolerant rather than judgmental, being committed to doing what is nourishing even if it is difficult, and being devoted to empowering other people with freedom and choice rather than taking their power away. This type of love may be fierce, but never hateful. It may be loud and insistent, but not manipulative. It will always seek the greatest good for everyone involved, constantly inventing ways to improve well-being and to relieve suffering.   Authentic compassion manages to be both boldly courageous and sincerely humble at the same time, always seeking ways to be strong while also being gentle and affectionate. And although we don't want to force Eilon to interact with others in some predefined way, or make him feel guilty if he isn't perfectly compassionate all the time, we can still nudge him in the right direction and hope for the best.

But what is the end result Eilon desires most? Well, in order for Eilon to be nourished at all, we need to find groups of people where we feel at home – where we aren't putting on some special act just to fit in. It is easy and natural to focus on being what other people expect of us, and that is what Eilon will sometimes do so that he can have a sense of belonging and community.   And to some extent, we all conform to society's roles and expectations in order to function in the world. However, a truly supportive community is defined by shared agreements that already exist below the surface of casual interactions. That is, when the deeper beliefs and values that we share with others are already in harmony, then we don't need to try as hard to fit in or get along.   And this is what Eilon really longs for.   Someone may like the same music I like, or enjoy the same activities, or even have similar cultural experiences, and these may seem like an easy way to connect with that person. But far more essential will be what they believe is truly important in life.   How do they define the purpose of their own existence? What value do they place on other people and relationships? Where do they find the most joy in each day? What ideas, principles or types of experience do they care most about? Where are their passions focused?   When we find people whose most dearly held beliefs and values resonate strongly with our own, not only can we begin creating a community that nurtures Eilon more fully, but become a resource for others to nourish themselves as well.

Conversations with Eilon

An interesting thing about Eilon is that, aside from his insistence that we socialize with like-hearted and like-minded people as often as possible, he won't have a lot to say to us directly. Instead, what informs us most about Eilon's needs is what we hear from those other people. He is constantly listening to others and reacting to what they say, so that is where we can discern a bit of initial guidance. What will help us most is exposing Eilon to as many different kinds of relationships as possible – in as many different situations and groups of people as possible – so that we can gather the broadest sampling of interactions to draw upon. This is one of those times when we have to learn from doing.

What kinds of relationships are there? Well, there are our closest, most intimate friendships. There are our romantic relationships. There is the family we grew up with.   There are groups of people we want to be around because they share our interests, values, ways of thinking or beliefs. There are relationships of convenience, like work relationships or fair-weather friends. And there are the strangers we meet on the street with whom we share an unspoken social contract – where we respect each other's physical space, don't pry too deeply into each other's personal life, try to be polite, and so on. And the more we interact in these different categories of relationship, the more information Eilon will have to work with – the more he will be able to convey to us what is most important and nourishing for him.

Three conclusions will rapidly become clear to us the more kinds of relationships we engage in each day. The first is that we need most if not all of these different kinds of relationships to grow and thrive. We might make do for a time with one or two types of connections that we feel are important, but we really can't rely on them to be fully nourished. No matter how close we feel to one or two people, they can never engage us on all the levels we need to thrive. Not only will Eilon be undernourished, but all of our other inner children as well, for relationships create the fertile earth for every kind of nurturing. At the same time, no matter how agreeable and safe a group of like-minded and like-hearted folks may seem at first, there will always be shifts and evolutions in us, or in other members of our community, that will temporarily interrupt our sense of acceptance and agreement. And this is the second conclusion: that healthy relationships are not static and do not stay the same forever, there will always be growth and change. The third conclusion is that those individuals or groups that endure the longest will be those with whom we share our most precious personal values, interests, ways of thinking and beliefs. These are the most critical to mutual well-being. It is also constructive to associate with people whose attitudes and habits are different from our own – who believe different things or value different things – just to keep things interesting, broaden our understanding of the world, and sharpen our minds. But we won't ever completely relax or be able to build deep bonds of trust unless there is more agreement than disagreement.

So all of these relationships are important, and our conversations with Eilon will mainly take place through our conversations and interactions with others. This is how we learn what Eilon needs, and what our personal supportive community will look and feel like. As we invite more and more relationships into our lives that agree with our values and connect with us on many different levels, we strengthen Eilon's ability to grow and evolve. Why? Because, by doing this, we create an interconnected web of enduring exchanges with other people, a loving community that encourages us to be true to ourselves even as we support others. And once again there is a balancing act: between becoming controlling or overly dependent on the one hand, and too detached and distant on the other; or between trying to fulfill everyone else's expectations and only caring about ourselves; or between feeling isolated and alone, and feeling overwhelmed or stretched too thin. If we can engineer that middle ground for ourselves, our connections with others will be strong and flexible.

Our instinct may be to seek a community of shared values that is already established – an existing organization, resource network, discussion group, activities group, etc. Sometimes, however, the only way we can experience a fellowship of likeminded people is to create that fellowship ourselves. By inviting people to get together to explore certain creative interests, spiritual interests, casual hobbies, etc. we can synthesize a new supportive community that benefits ourselves and others. For some of us this may feel a little scary at first, and it helps to have one or two established friends to get a group like this started, but the benefits almost always far outweigh the risks. And finally, another helpful tool for building a community of shared values is the Integral Coregroup. These are groups designed to explore Integral Lifework and support integral practice. They are described in detail in the "Our Partners in Parenting" chapter, and if you can't find an established on in your area, you could start one yourself.

Questions for Reflection & Discussion

- What does your supportive community currently look like? What are the personal values those relationships amplify?

- What sort of spoken or unspoken rules does your community have about what particular relationships should look, feel and sound like?

- What do you think the similarities are between a codependent relationship and a compassionate relationship? What are the differences?

- How do you recognize relationships where you can just "be yourself," in contrast to those where you are fulfilling the expectations of others, or acting out a fixed idea of some social role?

- Why do you think it might be important to connect with other people on many different levels or dimensions (emotional, mental, spiritual, etc.)?

- In your experience, has your surrounding culture encouraged you to search for happiness and contentment within yourself, or has it encouraged you to look outside of yourself for these things? In either case, why do you think this is so?

- What is the maximum number of people you think you could feel very close to? What is the minimum number you feel your Eilon requires to be nourished and sustained?

- What qualities and support do you feel you offer others in the course of your relationships with them?

- What is the most nurturing thing you could do for your Eilon in the next twenty-four hours?

LADA THE LOVER – FULFILLING SEXUALITY

"Lada" (lah-dah) is a Slavic name attributed to the ancient goddess of love, fertility and beauty. Lada is one of the most powerful children within, although most of the time she is so preoccupied with her various plans and strategies that she doesn't seem to realize how much power she has. Certainly all of the other children tend to watch her intently, wondering just what she will do next. Now Lada has this power for many different reasons. She is concerned first and foremost with making sure that the human species continues, so this alone gives her a lot of influence and authority. She is very stubborn about achieving this goal, and will say or do almost anything to make it happen. Usually she accomplishes her objectives with her irresistibly persuasive charm and promises of physical pleasure – promises she can actually deliver on fairly reliably. She is so stunningly beautiful it makes one's heart ache, and she is so charismatic that the natural inclination of everyone close to her is to go willingly and joyfully wherever she wishes. However, if all of her charms aren't successful, then she will resort to more extreme measures. She will lie, cheat, steal, manipulate, bully…whatever! She is exceedingly strong-willed, very persistent, and hardly ever sleeps.

Of course, Lada isn't only concerned with reproduction. She really likes having sex for its own sake, too. In fact she likes it so much that she will provide us with all sorts of reasons why we should have sexual experiences regularly, and maybe even pursue new types of experiences whenever we become bored with what we already have. This has sometimes gotten Lada in a bit of hot water regarding cultural rules and taboos around sex. This is because impulsive, excessive or seemingly indiscriminate sexual interactions with lots of new people can often be destructive to social expectations and social contracts. For example, some cultures believe that marriage means being sexually monogamous. In order to maintain the concept of a stable family structure in those cultures, sex outside of marriage is strongly discouraged. Most cultures find sexual intercourse between siblings to be genetically and morally risky, and many cultures outlaw any type of sexual interactions between children and adults, between humans and animals, and so on. If someone is perceived as having lots of sexual partners all the time, or having a stronger than usual sexual appetite, then they tend to be condemned or ridiculed within some cultures. And nearly all modern cultures place limits on sexual displays in public – whether it involves how much of the body our clothing is supposed to cover, or what kinds of sexual interactions are permissible in public view. And of course our sexual behaviors can also incur health risks, because of sexually transmitted diseases, which also tend to carry a strong cultural stigma. But it's important to realize that Lada really doesn't care about any of this. Not at all. She has no moral misgivings about gratifying her own needs – she just wants to have sex!

Alas, as with all of our other inner children, we just can't let Lada have her way all of the time. We need to find that middle ground between restricting or oppressing her into starving sadness, and letting her run completely out-of-control. Why? Because that is the most loving thing to do. Just as we explored creating healthy boundaries and discipline for Wachiwi, Manjit, Adelyte, Eilon and Luceria, we must do the same for Lada. If we always gave our children everything they wanted whenever they wanted it, they would become just as unhappy, unruly and unmanageable as if we gave them nothing at all. The secret to their enduring happiness is balance.

How do we achieve this with Lada? What constitutes a "balanced" amount of sexual excitement and gratification? Thankfully, we have some built-in helpers with this particular balancing act, and those are the various types of intimacy available to us. There is physical intimacy, which is about the comfortable closeness and openness between people's bodies. There is emotional intimacy, which is about the comfortable closeness and openness between people's emotional selves. You could say physical intimacy represents how easily and openly the Wachiwi (physical self) within me is willing to relate to the Wachiwi within you, and emotional intimacy represents how easily and openly my Adelyte (emotional self) can relate to your Adelyte. We can also include mental intimacy, too – how does my Manjit (mental self) relate to your Manjit? Do they get along? Is there a strong resonance or empathy between them? And there is spiritual intimacy, which defines how closely and openly my Shen (spiritual self) and your Shen can connect and relate.

Whenever there is some form of intimacy in play, it naturally regulates the intensity of Lada's sexual drive, and helps define boundaries for her willingness, curiosity, interests and satisfaction. Why? Because the more levels and types of intimacy that are made available between two people – intimacy of the heart, mind, spirit and body – the more easily sexual intimacy can be achieved, and the more sustained and satisfying sexual gratification will become over time. Without those other connections, the sexual act may be intensely exciting and pleasurable when it is new, but when the novelty fades so will the sense of satisfaction. With these other types of connection, sex is enhanced and expanded into a deeper interplay of emotions, thoughts, sensations and spirit. Lada may sometimes insist that sex without these intimacies can be fun – and that may be true – but short-term fun is not the same thing as long-term satisfaction.

And now we are beginning to see how the nourishment of each inner child directly influences the nourishment of every other. For if Manjit, Adelyte, Wachiwi and Shen aren't being fully nurtured, their unhappiness will interfere with Lada's sense of fulfillment, and influence how she believes she must go about getting fed. Likewise, when we neglect Lada's needs, that can interfere with nourishing our other dimensions as well. What we still need to figure out is just what level of fulfillment Lada requires to contribute her own energy to our overall well-being. And for that, we need to have a conversation with her.

Conversations with Lada

At first it might seem as though listening to our own body is enough to understand Lada's needs, but this is only part of the picture. For just as with Eilon, where we consulted with our community to understand how best to nourish him, with Lada we will also want to consult with our sexual partner to better understand how Lada's nourishment can unfold. When a partner is absent, Lada will of course make her presence known through our own sexual curiosity, interests and fantasies, and we can respond to her more directly. But whenever a partner is involved, that interaction is what will enhance Lada's nourishment, helping her contribute to our overall well-being. Whenever we honestly and openly communicate our sexual desires to our partner, and invite them to do the same, Lada can amplify her nourishment through that communication. Our desires include our sexual interests, favorite sensations, fantasies, wants, questions, excitements, curiosities, and so forth. Much of this communication may be expressed in non-verbal ways by each person, so it is important to pay attention to those cues. It might be a smile, a look, a touch, a sound...but Lada is there, making her needs known. Nevertheless, having an open, honest, relaxed, non-judgmental conversation with our partner about sex will strengthen Lada's confidence and ability to express herself.

How Lada relates to her siblings will also help us understand her better. Does she have a good relationship with Wachiwi? Is there frequent, open and honest communication between them? For example, can Wachiwi relax into Lada's sexual priorities, or does Wachiwi resist them or feel uncomfortable? Does Manjit respect and appreciate Lada's desires, or resent them and try to deprioritize Lada's needs? Has Shen introduced Lada to the spiritual aspects of sexuality, and has Lada been receptive to this? Does Lada respect and listen to her brothers and sisters, allowing their wants and needs to be met? Or does Lada insist that she always come first? Remember that Lada is very strong-willed, and sometimes will walk right over her siblings in pursuit of her goals. But when there is balance, harmony and mutual appreciation between all of our inner children, then it is much more likely they will all be equally and thoroughly understood, appreciated and cared for. This is why we must encourage Lada to be patient, compassionate and respectful of her siblings' needs, and to likewise encourage honesty and openness between all of our inner children.

Questions for Reflection & Discussion

- What has your relationship with Lada been like?   Do you feel you have balanced her priorities with those of your other inner children?

- Is Lada respectful and appreciative of her siblings?   Are they respectful and appreciative of her?

- Have you developed increasing levels of intimacy with a sexual partner – in mind, spirit, body and heart? How has that changed your sexual interactions with them?

- Are you able to speak openly, honestly and regularly with your sex partner about your sexual desires and theirs?

- Do you feel your sexual interests or activities are somehow judged by society? Why or why not?

- Has Lada ever persuaded you to do something you later regretted? Do you think she could do so again?

- Why do you think there are so many taboos around sex? Why is it sometimes a difficult subject to discuss with others?

- Do you have a fairly good awareness of Lada's needs from day-to-day? Can you hear her voice clearly? Is she able to be open and honest with you?

- Do you think it is productive to sometimes take a break from nourishing Lada?

- What is the most nurturing thing you could do for Lada in the next twenty-four hours?

Fabian the Gardner – Building a Legacy

"Fabian" (fay-bee-un) is a boy's name that has different meanings. On one hand it comes from the Latin word for *bean*, and possibly also relates to a Roman clan name meaning *grower of beans*. On the other hand it also implies caution, care and avoiding direct conflict when dealing with difficult circumstances – as was credited to the military strategy of Fabius Maximus in the second century B.C. As an inner child, Fabian is mostly interested in making your personal joys and passions available for other people in the future. That is, he wants to create a pleasurable legacy for future generations that is uniquely yours. He will approach this very practically and systematically, and often spend as much energy securing and protecting what you will leave behind for others as he does creating that legacy. Fabian is always looking to the future, and how that future can reflect some piece of who and what we are as a person. Among all of our children, he is one of the most pragmatic and cautious.

Unfortunately, many of us don't pay much attention to Fabian, and are unable to provide him what he needs to create and sustain this legacy. Why? Because we are often too caught up in the excitement of the present to listen to Fabian's quiet reminders. This can be tragic, because although he can be soft spoken and meek, his potential contribution to our well-being and development is immense. Many of humanity's greatest accomplishments are the result of Fabian's desire to engineer something meaningful and lasting for other people. What sorts of things does Fabian bring into being? Well, it could be anything. As long as it grows naturally from our inner passions and joys, it can evolve into lasting greatness. People's legacies range from the creative to the practical, from something we can hold in our hands to an idea that only remains in our minds, or even a lasting feeling that resides in our hearts. When someone recalls a friend who has passed on, what do they remember about them? That their friend was wise, perhaps, or that they made the tastiest pastries ever, or that they were a patient parent, or a good listener. And legacies aren't always things that are consciously remembered, either. Sometimes a legacy is a way of doing things, or a way of thinking about life, or a way of interacting with others that is unconsciously repeated by others without ever knowing where it came from.

But whatever our legacies may be, Fabian also takes special care to make sure that our joys and passions have a safe and secure environment where they can endure. In fact, he can sometimes become a little obsessed about this, so we have to be careful not to let him become so carried away with safety and security that we no longer have freedom to explore, experiment and share. For example, let's say your legacy happens to be making beautiful paper butterflies. Fabian might then insist that you go out and build a large concrete bunker, deep underground, to physically protect those butterflies from harm. Then he might insist you spend all your time down there so you can remain safe and secure. But living in a bunker all the time would be counterproductive to sharing your legacy with others! It would likely also interfere with the resources and inspiration required to create more butterflies. And this is how Fabian can sometimes sabotage himself. Once again we must strike a careful balance.

Now keep in mind that creating and securing a legacy can be very difficult to *do*; in fact it may be impossible to have a legacy at all if we are always preoccupied with *doing*. Legacies evolve out of what comes naturally for us, they blossom from who and how we naturally are in each moment. This is why Fabian works in the background much of the time. He watches our other inner children to see what they enjoy, then encourages them to pursue those interests, working in harmony to fashion something that will outlive them all. Even if Fabian's intuition picks up on any dangers to our legacy along the way, he will push us toward safety and security, or encourage us to be as consistent and reliable as possible, rather than confront us directly. That is just his nature – he treads very carefully and quietly within. Although Fabian may sometimes worry and fuss, he avoids being demanding or insistent; instead, he may just suffer silently and hope we will make better decisions moving forward. So Fabian is very cautious, but he isn't controlling.

Even though Fabian likes to work in the background, we still need to support and encourage him, and listen to his needs. We need to provide him with the building blocks of an enduring legacy so he doesn't become frustrated or depressed. Like all of our other inner kids, Fabian just wants to be loved. To help him, we need to create a garden where he can plant our legacy. If we create helpful conditions for Fabian to thrive, he will have a lot to share with us – and a lot to share with others. So our first step is actually to nourish all of our other inner children – that is the garden where our legacy will first take root. Then we just need to make room in our lives for Fabian to do his part, and listen for his voice.

Conversations with Fabian

So how can we maintain conditions that are helpful for Fabian's efforts? How can we secure an environment where Fabian can freely express his will and begin creating our legacy? There are several ways to do this. One of the first things we can do is make sure we have physical safety for ourselves and those we care about. Fabian is like a nervous kitten who runs and hides under a bed whenever there is a lot of fighting, angry yelling or disruption going on. He'll only venture out when he feels safe to do so. And we can encourage this sense of safety by making sure the people in our lives are not angry, argumentative, hostile sorts of people – and that we don't live or work in a community that is at war with itself. If we're living in a war zone, we'll probably have to wait until that war is over before we catch a glimpse of Fabian at all. But if we can sleep soundly in our beds without feeling threatened or worried, this will help Fabian flourish. As with any garden, we just can't have others running all over it, setting things on fire, trampling new plants, digging things up and so on. Our garden needs some peace and quiet to grow and flourish.

The second way we can help Fabian is to have a regular schedule of nourishment for other inner kids – at least most of the time. To eat, sleep, work and play at roughly the same times each day, and for the same length of time each day, will allow Fabian to interact with his siblings more easily, and help him understand what they are really the most passionate and joyful about. In other words, the very act of making sure that all our inner children's needs are met each day will itself encourage Fabian to engineer a legacy. If we are constantly interrupted, or always changing our plans, or never able to find a regular rhythm to our day or week, it will be hard for Fabian to find time and energy to complete his efforts. Using the garden analogy again, our life needs regular weeding, watering and harvesting. We can't just be random about these things and expect our garden to thrive.

The third way we can enhance Fabian's environment is by cultivating deep, loving and trusting relationships with other people – which is part of what Eilon will help us do as he cultivates a supportive community. Do we allow ourselves to share our passions and pleasurable experiences with others? Do our friends understand, encourage and assist our efforts? Do we feel like we can truly be ourselves around those who are part of our daily life? As Eilon would tell us, having plenty of friends and a strong supportive community will nourish us in many ways. And one way to measure how friendly and supportive others really are is how frequently and easily they encourage us in things we are passionate about or that we really enjoy. If all of the time we spend with others just depletes us and undermines or minimizes what we think is important, then we need to find some new people to hang out with. What if our closest friends picked and ate all our garden's beans without asking? What if they thought their own plantings were more important and insisted we help them water their garden all the time? What if they were never willing to help us with some much-needed weeding...? Then our garden wouldn't flourish very easily. We need to have people in our lives who are willing to kneel beside us in the dirt, to help us tend our plants at least as much as we help tend theirs.

And, finally, there is only so much time in the day, so much energy to accomplish a task, and so much of any one resource to draw upon to enable our legacy. This means we must be clear about our priorities, about what we value most and what we think is the most important use of our time. Even though our other inner children compete for our attention in these areas, this is where Fabian really shines. Because he understands exactly what is most important to us as a whole person – as a sum of all those different inner voices and needs – and if we create space in our lives for him to come out into the daylight, Fabian will help clarify these priorities. This kind of clarity will take time to rise up into our awareness, but as we let go of urgently *doing* and relax into more balanced *being*, the nature of our legacy will become obvious, and Fabian's voice will be more clearly heard.

How does a perfectly balanced existence happen? It happens when all of our inner children feel secure that they will be nurtured and appreciated. When they can relax, then we can relax, and Fabian can find the common ground – the unified and harmonized effort of all our passions and enjoyments – that leads us to an enduring legacy. Our inner garden will grow because we let all of it grow together; because we don't try to harvest things before they are ripe, or obsessively water one section to the neglect of another, or constantly plant new things before we've harvested the last planting's growth. Fabian is a great gardener. He will help us understand how to best utilize the soil of our inner life if we provide him the space, time, relationships and resources to do so.

Questions for Reflection & Discussion

- What has your relationship with Fabian been like?   Has the shape and nature of your own personal legacy risen up to the surface?

- What are some of the legacies of others that you have observed or experienced?

- How do you think you can best transition from *doing* things you enjoy and are passionate about to a sense of *being* those things?

- Do you find it easy to create and keep schedules for nourishing yourself regularly in every dimension? Why or why not?

- Do you feel your surrounding environment and relationships support your passions and interests? Why or why not?

- Does your current lifestyle provide the safety and stability required to encourage Fabian's success? Why or why not?

- Why is it sometimes necessary to weed our legacy-garden?

- What is the most nurturing thing you could do for Fabian in the next twenty-four hours?

PEACEFUL IRINA – ALL ABOUT REMEMBERING

"Irina" (ee-ree-nuh) is a Slavic name that means *peace*. And Irina can be one of the most powerful forces for both inner peace and its expression in a peaceful life. She wants to be peaceful, but she can also be very disruptive, too. Experiencing one outcome or the other depends on how we decide to interact with her. The reason Irina is so influential is because she is the keeper of all our memories. She has every memory in a little box that she can open whenever she wants. If your Irina spends a lot of time opening boxes that are sad or upsetting, all of your inner children are probably going to end up feeling sad or upset much of time. If she opens memory boxes where you did well, or achieved your goals, or helped others, then you are much more likely to do well, achieve your goals and continue helping others. It's very strange and mysterious how our memories help determine how we are from moment-to-moment, but if we have a good relationship with Irina, we will shape how that mystery unfolds.

One thing to remember about Irina is that she will always be opening those memory boxes whether we want her to or not – and whether we are aware of it or not. We may want to ignore certain memories, or make them seem less important, but Irina knows that all memories are important, and will keep opening boxes and looking at them over and over again. She can't help it. This is sort of game for her. "What will I take a peek at today?" she says to herself, rubbing her hands together with gleeful anticipation. For Irina, it doesn't really matter whether one memory is shocking, another frustrating, another pleasurable and another exhilarating…for her, each memory is valuable in itself. So there are no "good" or "bad" memories for Irina, there is just an endless pile of boxes and a continuous sense of fascination and discovery. But if we can help her be a bit less compulsive, and instead be a little more thoughtful about her memory box selection, we can encourage peace and harmony rather than discord in our inner world.

Why is it important to do this? Well, because the story of our present is made up of our past. We cannot separate who we are in the present from all that we have been before. Our memory shapes the tendencies, thoughts and behaviors of all of our inner children. To fully appreciate and nurture them, we need to explore our memory as carefully and caringly as we can. As just one example, it is often the case that our ideas about our natural strengths and weaknesses are formed by certain events from our past. Did we succeed well at some activities when we were young? Did we fail at others? Did someone important in our life treat us in ways that made us believe we were talented in some areas and hopelessly unskilled in others? These experiences will influence how we view our own competencies now – even though we may have changed, learned or grown in ways that altered those competencies over time. Another example is that we learned how to interact with others – friends, strangers, family, authority figures – when we were little. In the present, we tend to imitate how we were treated and how we observed others were treated as we were growing up. And, perhaps most important of all, we learned how to care for ourselves by the examples of caring and kindness we experienced as a child. How we were cared for is how we instinctively continue to take care of ourselves. So all of these memories contribute to our current understanding of who we are, how we should act, and what healthy and nourishing self-care looks like.

Conversations with Irina

There are many ways we can interact with Irina, and the following exercise is just one of them. Give it a try and see what you think. In this example, you are showing Irina a compassionate way to look into her collection of memory boxes. You aren't telling her what to do, exactly, you are just showing her what any caring and responsible parent would do for their child. As with all such exercises, it is helpful to set your intention before you begin by feeling and saying, "May this be for the good of All."

Find a place to sit where things will be quiet and undisturbed for about twenty minutes. Sit comfortably with your eyes closed, breathing deeply and regularly. Briefly focus your attention various muscles all in your body – your shoulders, neck, forearms, calves, stomach and so on – and imagine each one relaxing and softening. Do this for five minutes or so, until you feel as relaxed as possible.

Now imagine you are sitting in a circular room with a high ceiling, with doors regularly spaced along the circular wall. If you can, try to color the walls a soft peach or pale pink color, and the doors as white with gold knobs on them. The floor could be wood or marble or some other kind of natural material.

Behind each white door with a gold knob is a scene from your past. Without opening the door, begin preparing a scene behind one of the doors that involved you directly when you were a young child, and created strong emotions in you at that time – it could be fear, or guilt, or anger, or confusion…it doesn't matter as long as the emotions were strong. Now just know that the scene is there behind the door, without necessarily visualizing it completely. Perhaps you might hear what is going on through the door, or merely anticipate what you will find there. Keep breathing regularly and try to relax. The door will not open until you are ready.

When you are ready, approach the door. Feel the gold handle in your hand. Listen for a moment and prepare yourself for what you are about to see. Keep breathing regularly and try to relax. Now open the door and look at what is happening. Perhaps you will see the scene you expected. Perhaps you will see something else. Just go with the flow of whatever you discover inside, and remain in the doorway. Know that you are safe and let yourself feel whatever emotions want to arise.

When you are ready, enter the scene beyond the door and look around until you find your younger self in that scene. Get as close as possible to your younger self and try to get their attention. Sometimes they may be very emotional, or want to turn away, or be preoccupied with what is happening in the scene…whatever state your younger self is in, just be a presence beside them.   Offer them your calm, caring, wise, adult companionship.

Once you are able to get your younger self's attention (by catching their eye with a gesture, speaking to them, touching their shoulder, or whatever way you can), hold out your arms to offer them a hug. Whatever happens next, keep breathing, remain as calm as possible, and be patient. If your younger self runs into your arms, hug them tight. If they just want to hold your hand, then let them do that. If they just want to talk to you, then have a conversation with them. Perhaps they'll have some questions for you, or the may be an opportunity for you to explain why there is nothing here for them to feel guilty or ashamed about. Whatever their actions or emotions – sadness, anger, panic, fear, laughter, excitement – just let their energy wash over you and be a comforting, stable, calm and caring presence for them.

If others in the scene begin to interact with you, gently disengage from them and focus on your younger self. You may have to ask these others to leave if they won't leave you alone. You want to spend time with your younger self right now, focusing all of your attention on them and no one else.

At a point when your younger self is calm and comforted, and when you have established positive and warm interaction with them, look into their eyes and tell them from your heart: "I will always be here for you. I love you. You can always count on me." Give them some time to absorb this. Repeat the words if necessary, and do your best to really mean them.

And finally, tell your younger self that you have only a few minutes remaining before you have to go, and let them decide what they want to do with the rest of your time together. Assure them that you will be back soon. Spend those last few minutes being encouraging and reassuring. Then exit the scene by the white door through which you entered, and return to the circular room. Be sure to close the door behind you.

Open your eyes and reflect on your experience for a few minutes.
Perhaps capture some thoughts in your journal. Being true to your
word, try this exercise again another day, maybe with a different
memory in mind, but always returning to some version of your younger
self. By doing this once or twice a week, work through different kinds
of experiences – those that caused strong emotions that were both
positive and negative for your younger self.

When you do this sort of exercise, you are showing Irina what is most
important to you, and that will help her prioritize her efforts too. She
won't just be opening random boxes out of excitement, or boxes that
remind her of something you happen to be doing, or boxes she just
happens to think are interesting…she'll start to open boxes that support
how you consciously want to be towards your younger self from
moment-to-moment. She'll want to help you be a kind and
compassionate parent with all of the memories she provides.

What kinds of childhood experiences should you revisit? I think it is
important to be as diverse as possible in our remembering, to provide
Irina with the most flavorful and interesting nourishment possible.
There should be memories that make us feel powerful, and memories
that make us feel weak. Memories that are full of fear, and memories full
of joy. Memories that filled us with guilt and shame when we were little,
and memories that filled us with tranquility and contentment. Memories
that are painful, and memories that are funny. Most importantly, we
should try to recall memories that involve our parents, family members
and early childhood friends, because these are more likely to contain the
strongest associations and life lessons that inform us in the present.

Questions for Reflection & Discussion

- What has your relationship with Irina been like? Have you been open to memories she shares with you, or have you shied away from certain memories or from parts of your past?

- Can you tell how memories of your past have shaped who you are today? Are there pattern of emotion, or types of relationship, that existed in your childhood and seem to be repeating themselves in the present?

- Are there certain memories that are particularly powerful for you? Or ones that keep showing up unexpectedly, even when you are thinking of other things? Is there one memory in particular that seems representative of how your life has unfolded for you?

- Can you imagine using the exercise in this chapter to help reprocess, reprioritize, understand or heal a potent memory from your past? Why or why not?

- Are there any memories or periods of your life that you are nervous or anxious about examining? Why or why not?

- Do you think it is ever a good idea not to dwell on certain memories, even if they are happy ones? Why or why not?

- What is the most nurturing thing you could do for Irina in the next twenty-four hours?

ASIM THE GUARDIAN – WHAT WE THINK ABOUT OURSELVES

"Asim" (ah-seem) is an Arabic name that means *protector* or *defender*. Among our children, Asim can often be the fiercest and most serious. Asim spends much of his time gazing outward into the world, always on alert for possible dangers or surprises, intent on protecting his siblings from any and all harm. However, Asim should also be spending some time looking inward, to understand and appreciate what it is he is protecting. Imagine a soldier who is always on alert at the battlefront of some distant land. No matter how fiercely loyal and patriotic he wants to be, if he never returns to his homeland, he will forget why he is fighting, and who and what he is fighting for. He will forget what "homeland" really means to him. This is Asim's Achilles' Heel (his greatest weakness), and our job as his parent is to gently help him overcome it.

There are many ways to help Asim look inward, and we have already explored some of them in previous chapters. The key to all of them is being able to peer inside ourselves without blinking or flinching, always trying to be kind, patient and accepting about what we find there. The challenge with Asim is that he really doesn't want to look at all. It's not in his nature. He is convinced that his role – his entire purpose – is to be on-guard against the threats, worries and unexpected changes from the outside world. For him, spending time looking inward seems like a silly and dangerous risk. But, as with our other inner kids, we need to help him realize there is a more balanced way to go about defending his family. If we can encourage him to turn some of his vigilance inward, we will help him realize that trying to better understand that inner life is essential to protecting it.

What is Asim really all about? He is about survival. Asim is obsessed with helping us be as effective as possible in navigating the world in which we live. His protectiveness is a deep-rooted concern for our very existence, and he is always looking for ways to improve our situation. If Asim believes we are effective at surviving and thriving, then he will feel pretty good about things, and will help us feel good about who we are as a person. If Asim is full of doubt and fear about our ability to succeed in life, then his paranoia will erode our sense of well-being and the confidence we have in any of our abilities. So another part of our parental responsibility is to reassure Asim that he is doing a good job protecting us, and that we continue to be capable and self-assured in our day-to-day survival because of his efforts. We need to be brave and steadfast in our love for Asim and our confidence in his abilities, knowing that, as long as we support and nurture him, he will learn whatever he needs to learn in order to protect us and help us succeed.

Conversations with Asim

To summarize, then, Asim needs to appreciate what he is protecting, he needs to understand how best to protect it, and he needs to believe he is doing a good job. One way we can touch on all of these areas at once is by regularly completing a brief inventory of how we are caring for all our inner children, as well as how we will refine and expand that care over time. For Asim, the well-being of our inner family is the strongest evidence of our overall success in life. The healing, harmony and growth of our inner kids reassures Asim that he is doing his part. Below are some questions that will help Asim appreciate the current state of our inner family. Later on in the book there is another exercise – the seven-day nourishment assessment – which can be used to expand on these questions and further connect with Asim.

Just as with previous inner conversation techniques, first create some quiet space and time to reflect on each of the following questions. As with all such exercises, it is helpful to set your intention before you begin by saying, "May this be for the good of All," and feeling that intention in your heart as sincerely as possible. Sit comfortably with your eyes closed, breathing deeply and evenly, and hold each of the following questions lightly in your mind. Avoid writing anything down for now. Just keep breathing and resting in silent awareness of whatever arises within you. When you have completed one run-through of the questions below, go back to the beginning and start over again, this time spending a little more time resting in whatever arises within you as a response to each question. When you have completed the second review of the questions, try writing down your reflections and conclusions – so you have a record and can compare them to future reflections over time.

- Do I feel I take good care of myself? Why or why not?

- Do I feel safe and secure most of the time, or do I feel vulnerable or afraid? What are some of the reasons I might feel this way?

- Am I my own person, with my own vision for my life, or am I still in a power struggle with my parents, my siblings or other people around me? Am I confidently steering my own life, or am I still trying to establish my direction and independence?

- Do I show the "real me" to the world, with all my warts and weaknesses, or do I put on an act to protect myself? Am I secure and confident in who I am, or am I always trying to be what someone else expects me to be?

- Do I have a lasting sadness in my heart about things that I have lost? If so, why is that?

- Do I still feel guilt over something I did in the past, or have I fully forgiven myself? If I still feel guilt, why haven't I forgiven myself?

- Do I believe I have a purpose in this life, and that I am fulfilling that purpose?

- Am I always honest with those I love about everything I think and do? Why or why not?

- Do I follow through on whatever I commit to doing? Why or why not?

- Do I live my life according to clear personal values and goals? Why or why not?

- Do I have a genuine connection with my spiritual self? Do I regularly experience a close relationship with the spiritual aspects of my being?

- Do I love myself? Do I really care about my own well-being? Do I want to be whole and thrive? Why or why not?

- Do I enjoy life to its fullest every day? Why or why not?

- Am I surrounded by people who want the best for me, and who connect with my beliefs, interests and values? Do my friends and loved ones support and encourage the vision I have for my life?

- Do I have a satisfying sex life? Do I enjoy sex? Am I a caring and skillful lover?

- Am I a playful person? Do I have a playful sense of humor? Do I frequently laugh at myself? Can I chuckle about my quirks or mistakes when someone points them out to me?

- As a result of all of my actions and interactions with others, would I leave a positive influence and legacy behind if I vanished tomorrow? Why or why not?

- Am I able to really relax and let go in stressful situations? Why or why not?

- Do I have genuine affection for my own body? Do I believe my habits and attitudes have a positive influence on my body's overall health and appearance? Why or why not?

- Am I a creative and imaginative person? Do I regularly express myself in creative ways?

- Do I appreciate the creative efforts of others? Do I regularly expose my senses to the arts? Do I stimulate my imagination? Why or why not?

- Do I keep my mind sharp and alert? Do I keep it fed with new and interesting information and experiences? Do I regularly stimulate my brain? Why or why not?

Answers to these questions can be revealing. They can show us that Asim has a lot to be proud of and should feel good about what he is protecting and how he is protecting it – maybe even some strengths or skills we didn't realize we had. And the answers can also reveal some stumbling blocks to Asim's strength and confidence. They may show us some unattractive things that we can easily change, or weaknesses that we may not be able to change so easily. Whatever is revealed, we eventually need to embrace all of these strengths and weaknesses as part of who we are. We must learn to love and cherish everything about ourselves. We don't need to judge ourselves too harshly at one extreme, or puff ourselves up with arrogance at the other extreme. Instead, if we can relax and let go of both judgment and overconfidence, we can eventually fall in love with our whole self...just as we are, without needing to condemn ourselves or inflate our ego.

Yet how do we do this? How can we learn to love ourselves unconditionally? It takes practice. In a way, the whole process of getting to know our inner children, understanding their needs, and discovering the best ways to nourish and support them is really all about learning to loving ourselves. It takes time, practice, courage and careful attention to master this process. But eventually, even though we may stumble and struggle on occasion, we will become kind, caring and forgiving of all our quirks and foibles; we will recognize that just having awareness about them can help us better nourish ourselves, better navigate the world around us, and help Asim and all our other inner children thrive. And, eventually, we will also begin utilizing all of our strengths and talents to better nourish ourselves as well, feeling confident and happy about how we care for our inner family, and confident and happy in what we think about ourselves.

Questions for Reflection & Discussion

- What has your relationship with Asim been like?   Has he been a good protector and defender?   Why or why not?

- Has Asim been willing to look deep within you to better understand what he is protecting?

- What did the questions in this chapter reveal about Asim's role in your life?

- Do you think Asim can sometimes become too protective? Why or why not?

- Are there things you have discovered about yourself that you don't particularly like? If so, do you think you can become more accepting of those things? Or would you rather change them? Why or why not?

- How do you think all of your inner children may contribute to your sense of who you are? To your identity as a person?

- How often do you think do you think it would be beneficial to consult with your inner kids? Daily? Weekly? Hourly?

- What is the most nurturing thing you could do for Asim in the next twenty-four hours?

TRUSTWORTHY NOBUKO – KEEPING PROMISES WITH YOURSELF

"Nobuko" (no-boo-koh) is a Japanese girl's name. Because it can be written different ways in Japanese, it may mean different things, but most of these meanings have to do with *faith, truth* and *fidelity*. Nobuko is the sort of child whose mere presence will keep us honest. Whenever we invent a story to cover up a mistake or avoid some sort of embarrassment, Nobuko will gaze into our eyes and stop us short, even as the words of a lie are forming on our lips. And she always knows when we are being dishonest...even if we are only lying to ourselves. That is her gift. Nobuko is fiercely committed to doing what is honorable and just. She also wants to hold us accountable for whatever we say we are going to do. In a moment of excitement we might exclaim to a friend, "Oh yes! I'm going to go to that party. I'll see you there!" Well, Nobuko will try to remind us of those words over and over again, so that we don't forget to follow through. And if we don't go to the party, we'd better have a good reason, or Nobuko will give us a stern talking-to. Even when we promise something out of guilt, or a desire to please someone, even when we commit on impulse and without thinking to some course of action, Nobuko will hold us accountable for the promises we make and the intentions we express. She is kind of a perfectionist about this. So if we want to nourish Nobuko, we must learn to carefully consider what we say, feel, think and do.

Nobuko can also help us distinguish between different kinds of honesty, and help us become diligent in each area. There is emotional honesty, which reflects how sincere and accurate our feelings and attitudes are from moment to moment. For example, am I really grateful that I received a certain gift, or am I just expressing gratitude out of sense of obligation? Am I really sad about someone being caught in an embarrassing situation, or do I actually think it's kind of funny? Then there is intellectual honesty, which examines whether we are really convinced of certain facts, or have sound reasons for thinking the way we do about someone or something. For example, I may assume something bad about a person because I heard some of my friends gossiping about them. But are my assumptions true? Or maybe I want to believe that aliens have visited Earth, so I collect lots of evidence to support that view, and ignore any information that exposes flaws in my reasoning. Then there is values honesty. Do I really believe getting a formal education is important? Or that people who steal should be thrown in jail? Do I really think being honest is important? And so on. There are actually many different kinds of honesty, but they all boil down to how aware we are about where our knowledge, perceptions and reactions come from, and how accurate they are. And, if we allow her to, Nobuko can help us develop this awareness.

Within our inner family, Nobuko also has another function. She wants all of her siblings to work in harmony with one another. For her, this is the clearest evidence that every inner child is following through on their commitment to every other child. This inner harmony is what "just and honorable" looks like to Nobuko. If everyone is working towards the same mutually-agreed-upon goal, supporting each others' efforts and cooperating to make sure everyone else within is equally nourished, this provides Nobuko with a lot of satisfaction. Outside of the family, Nobuko wants to encourage the same sort of harmony and cooperation as well. With other people, with other communities and nations, with the Earth and all its natural systems, with the spiritual realm, even with the Universe itself! She longs for there to be a healthy, mutually supportive balance in all arenas of being. She longs for there to be harmony, peace and mutual support between all aspects of existence.

She is also concerned with how responsibly we act in society, for this comes from the same place as her wanting us to be honest with ourselves. We learn much about how to perceive, feel, think and act from our family, community, culture and so on. As part of this, we learn to do things like follow laws, be considerate of others, vote if we live in a democracy, be generous when we see someone in need, and so on. We learn to participate and cooperate in society, so that we can be part of that society. These can be things we consciously agree with, or things that become habits without our being completely aware of them. For example, if we live in a culture that has certain expectations of its citizens, Nobuko will want us to fulfill those expectations unless we have a compelling reason not to. To wear clothes in public, for instance, or not cut into a line of waiting people, or not interrupt someone when they are speaking. It doesn't matter if we don't always agree with the social expectations of our society, because we are benefiting from everyone else trying to meet those expectations. Our own peace, safety and prosperity depends on everyone else following the same rules. So, according to Nobuko, it is our responsibility to follow those rules as well. Once again, this may relate to something as casual as being polite to an elderly person, or something as grave as not committing a violent crime. This is what mutual respect looks and feels like to Nobuko.

Of course, if some social expectation is really distasteful to our conscience and somehow seems fundamentally wrong to us, then Nobuko will want us do what we think is right and just and honorable in our own mind and heart. That is, what we believe is for the good of All, rather than what society seems to expect. She does not mean to be inflexible (though sometimes she can seem that way), she just wants us to be thinking about all of this, and to act as consistently as possible according to our personal values. Consistency is a really big deal to Nobuko, because if we act consistently, and speak consistently, and think consistently, there is a much higher likelihood we will have honesty and integrity in our actions, words, thoughts and feelings. However, some of the most challenging choices we often make are between what society expects, and what we think is right for ourselves and our loved ones. For Nobuko, that choice will always be about sticking to what we treasure most – and so we must become clear about what our most important priorities really are.

When we add all of these things together, the basic idea that Nobuko wants us to understand is that we need to follow through on mutually loving and respectful actions, in every situation, for the benefit of our own well-being and everyone else in society. This is what Nobuko might call "having integrity in all things." Ideally, this integrity should flow naturally out of compassion for ourselves and others. Feeling affection and love for everyone and everything is the preferred foundation for Nobuko's sense of fairness and justice. But even if our affection and caring is lacking in a certain situation, Nobuko still wants us to maintain integrity in all things. Even when it is really hard, or demands personal sacrifice, or even results in personal pain, she will insist that we maintain our best intention, attention and efforts to follow-through in every situation. Whatever the cost, she yearns for harmony, cooperation and mutual benefit for the good of All. This is the heart of Nobuko's just and honorable mindset.

Conversations with Nobuko

A helpful starting point in our conversations with Nobuko is to ask ourselves: "What is most important to me in this moment?" If we keep checking in on this throughout the day, being as honest as we can about it, we will begin to engage Nobuko in her favorite territory. Eventually, once we gain a clearer picture of what is really most important to us, we can ask a follow-up question: "Am I thinking, feeling, dreaming and acting in accordance with what is most important to me?" The answer to this question is Nobuko's primary obsession. She wants us to align our thoughts, feelings, dreams and actions with our innermost priorities. Only then will she be satisfied. So delving deeply and regularly into these two questions will open us up to Nobuko's voice.

However, one challenge we will have with Nobuko is finding the middle ground between two extremes. On the one hand, we don't want to ignore her and live dishonestly or without integrity. On the other, we don't want to allow Nobuko's obsession with honesty and integrity to become more important than love itself. That is, we don't want to become so rigid and rules-oriented that we forget that harmony and balance are supposed to flow from authentic kindness and compassion. At one extreme, we can't trust ourselves to do what is right, fair and just. And at the other extreme, we can't trust ourselves to do what is loving and kind. We want to support Nobuko and demonstrate that we respect her desire for integrity, but we can't allow that need to become more important than anything else. After all, she is just one of our inner children – no less important and no more important than any other. The following exercise is meant to help Nobuko appreciate the middle ground between these two extremes, and to honor her contribution to our well-being. As with all such exercises, it is helpful to set your intention before you begin by feeling and saying, "May this be for the good of All," and to feel that intention sincerely in your heart.

As a starting point you can begin each day by looking at yourself in the mirror – right into your eyes – and reciting the following affirmations one after the other. Try to summon as much courage and belief in these statements as you can when speaking them aloud, and pause for several breaths between each one to let it penetrate deeply into your mind, heart, body and soul. When you do this, you are inviting Nobuko into the forefront of your thoughts and intentions, and allowing her to hold you accountable. As you say each phrase aloud and think about what it means, you are testing your own resolve to be a good parent to Nobuko and nourish her with your words and actions. You are encouraging yourself to be completely, openly and humbly honest, and are asking Nobuko to help you achieve a consistent way of being.

"Because I am devoted to my own well-being, I seek understanding in my soul."

"As I come to know my soul, my heart brims to overflowing with compassionate affection."

"Because this love overflows my heart, my mind seeks a way to share it with others and let it expand into everything around me."

"Because my mind discerns the way, I express the boundless love of my heart and the deep understanding of my soul through every action."

"Because I trust in these intentions without reservation or doubt, I let go of the importance of my own involvement."

"Because I let go of my own importance, the effectiveness of my love is miraculous."

At the end of each day, just before you go to sleep, reflect back over your day to measure how these affirmations played out in your thoughts, feelings, actions and interactions. Did you exercise honesty and integrity in all things? Did you have consistent intention, attention and follow-through in each of them? Do you think Nobuko is pleased with how things went? Why or why not? If there are any areas that seem to present challenges for you, consider spending the next day focusing your attention on just those areas, always trying to balance honesty and integrity with kindness and affection. In this way we allow Nobuko to participate in our well-being and encourage harmony and peace within and without. We open the door for her to remind us of what integrity, honor and respect look like, while at the same time remembering that compassionate affection remains our most important motivation. For the good of All does not flow from rules, respect and honesty alone, but from a loving kindness that guides us into what is most just and honorable in-the-moment. At the same time, if we do not follow through on what we say we will do, or conform to the laws and expectations of society that our conscience agrees with, then we will not be able to love very effectively at all.

Questions for Reflection & Discussion

- What has your relationship with Nobuko been like? Have you allowed her to enhance your awareness about the honesty of your thoughts, feelings, words and actions?

- Why do you think Nobuko cares so much about being honest and following through on what you say you will do?

- Are there times when your Nobuko would be okay with lying in some way?

- How can we know when we are being emotionally dishonest with ourselves or someone else?

- What kinds of social expectations are you aware of in your culture? How do you feel about them? Do you think they are equally beneficial to everyone?   Do they agree with your personal values? Why or why not?

- Do you have a sense of what the balance looks and feels like between being rigid or rules-oriented, and being compassionate and kind? Why or why not?

- Do you feel like all your inner children get along? Do they work well and play well together? Why or why not?

- Why do you think harmony and peace – both within you and
  around you – is so attractive and important to Nobuko? How do
  you feel integrity, harmony and peace relate to each other?

- What is the most nurturing thing you could do for Nobuko in
  the next twenty-four hours?

PURPOSEFUL PEMBA – WHY ARE WE HERE?

"Pemba" (pehm-bah) has many different meanings, and can be a girl's or boy's name depending on the African or Tibetan culture where it is being used. I would like to refer the name Pemba here without any particular gender in mind. Pemba is concerned with one thing, and that is our life's meaning and purpose. Pemba is always asking the same sorts of questions in every situation: "Why am I here?" "What does this mean for my life?" "What is my purpose?" "Where will this lead me?" "How will I get there?" What Pemba desires more than anything is that our inner family knows with complete clarity where our ship-of-self is sailing, and that our ship always stays on course.

There are three critical pieces to being a good parent to Pemba. The first is clearly defining some sort of guiding vision for our life. What do we want our future to hold for us? What do we want to work towards in the short and long term? However we imagine our lives will eventually look and feel becomes is our guiding vision. Now we can arrive at this vision in many different ways – some of them conscious and deliberate, and others unconscious or accidental. But the key contributors to our guiding vision are simply what we value most. What do we feel is most important? What are we most passionate about? Is one thing more or less important than something else? Why do we feel this way? These are the kinds of questions that will inform our purpose.

The second critical skill for parenting Pemba is understanding how to enact our guiding vision and make it real. How will we go about expressing what we value most? What steps must we take to get from where we are now to where we want to be? What skills will we require? What resources will we need? What people, materials and environments will support our vision? How will we maintain our energy and passion along the way? In this way we can plan how our vision will become reality. We may have many different plans over time, as we try one thing and then another to reach our goals. In fact we may even adjust the shape and feel of our vision from time to time, and therefore adjust our plans in response. But all the while we are thinking "What can I do today to reach the end result I imagine for my life...?"

The third parenting skill we must cultivate is to continually check on our progress, measuring what is actually happening against our original vision and all our plans. It wouldn't make much sense to continue with the same strategy if it isn't leading us closer to our goal, right? So we must constantly and carefully observe whether our actions and plans align with what we value most, what we believe to be important, and what seems the most meaningful. Do we remain passionate and committed about our life's vision over time? Do we still think the same things are most important? Is our life progressing as we hoped? Are we making our vision real in some way each and every day? Are we doing what we love to do, living the life we love to live, and being the person we love to be...?

What we are accomplishing when we nourish Pemba is nurturing our own personal will – that is, our individual energy that translates the impulses, wishes and yearnings from every dimension of our being into concrete actions. That individual energy is a constant, always ebbing and flowing within us, and if we don't consciously apply it somewhere, it will always find a way to express itself. Often, if we do not carefully consider our purpose, or if we choose a purpose that is somehow contrary to what our inner children really think is best or most appropriate for us, the energy of our will can actually cause us to become unbalanced, confused or seriously ill. This can happen to varying degrees with any of our inner kids, but Pemba in particular can unintentionally cause a lot of pain and suffering if this inner child remains on an unproductive, visionless path for too long.

What, then, is the best compass for this journey? Well, it is easy to look outside of ourselves for direction. What our parents think is important, or what they feel we should do, can have a strong influence on us. In the same way, our friends, educators and mentors, a business we work for, our religious community – all sorts of folks may have strong opinions about what is meaningful, what we should value most, and where our life should lead. And there will always be plenty of well-meaning people who will offer us guidance about all of this, too. Sometimes these influences and guidance can inspire us to explore things we never would have thought to explore, and that may be an important part of our overall education. However, it is also easy to get caught up in someone else's guiding vision, especially if they happen to be very driven or inspired when we are not. This is because Pemba's need for meaning and purpose is so strong. And once we are immersed in someone else's vision, that substitution of purpose can distract us from our own destination longer than is healthy or wise.

So really the best compass for our life's meaning and purpose is within us. As we explore what is most important to our inner children, our life's vision will become increasingly clear. If we create space and time for this inner compass to guide us, it will help Pemba chart our course and keep the rest of our inner family focused and united in harmony toward a shared vision. Pemba knows that all of these steps are essential nourishment. But unless we actively take part in the process, it is easy to forget why we are here and what is most important to us, and end up neglecting or even avoiding Pemba's promptings to live a meaningful and purposeful life.

Conversations with Pemba

In order for Pemba to gain clarity about our life's meaning and vision, we will probably need to take a break from our routine and exit our usual environment for a while. This might mean a few days alone in Nature, or a retreat with others who want to intuit their purpose in silent meditation, or keeping ourselves somewhere far away from the influences of work, friends, family and so on. It may require several such retreats to fully appreciate our purpose. But in each of these situations, we must look within ourselves. That is where all the answers lie.

I call the following exercise *dowsing for Light*. It is best suited as a sitting meditation, but could also be undertaken as a walking meditation for someone more comfortable doing it that way. It will probably need to be practiced several times – and in conjunction with the other exercises in this book – in order to have benefit. As with all such exercises, it is helpful to set your intention before you begin by feeling and saying, "May this be for the good of All."

First, create an inviting space within yourself. Sit or walk somewhere quiet where you won't be disturbed, take ten deep, slow breaths, and relax your whole being. Wipe your heart and mind clean of "must haves" and "have tos" and "can't dos" that are all wrapped up in the past and the future. Just empty yourself of all of that mess and pay attention to what is going on right now. If distracting thoughts or emotions arise just watch them arise and let them go. There is no reason to hold onto them. Allow yourself to become an empty stage where anything could happen...something ridiculous, or terrifying, or hilarious, or fascinating...anything. As a matter of setting your intention, try to avoid rejecting or resisting what you encounter, and allow any and all possibilities to occur.

Now crank open your intuitive faucet, and let it flow. With your attention directed inward, ask "What is my purpose?" Hold out the bowl of your consciousness to catch the stream of insights, sensations, images and ideas that arise. Let that flow accumulate in your mind and heart without trying to shape it or change it, and without turning off the source. Keep asking the question "What is my purpose?" Try not to edit or grasp onto what comes up, and don't worry about writing it down or remembering what you encounter. Just keep going, keep asking and searching and letting the flow continue. Breathe deeply and evenly and open yourself wide to the experience. Somewhere in that upwelling of ideas, sensations and images is a true reflection of who you are and what your life is about in this moment. You will recognize this event when you experience it. You will feel its certainty and rightness. You will sense its brightness and intensity. You will want to linger there to absorb its warmth. And you will feel both content and inspired because it has bubbled to the surface within you.

Keep the doors of your heart and mind open, your attention focused inward, and your breathing even for at least twenty minutes. As you develop greater concentration with practice, you might want to focus your attention inward for an hour or more. As you go deeper, you can begin to refine your vision with additional questions. "How will I express or accomplish this?" "What resources will assist me in my efforts?" "What specific outcomes should I plan for in the upcoming weeks?" Really, you can ask anything you want about how to fulfill your purpose. The key is to keep asking, remaining open, and letting whatever arises from within stream lightly across your receptive mind and heart. The answers may be very specific or more general, and sometimes it may take a while – days, weeks or even months – for you to fully understand what you encounter. As you gain more clarity about that meaning and importance, it can be helpful to capture your thoughts in a journal so you can return to them later.

This dowsing for Light practice is just a first step. The next part of nourishing Pemba – and thereby living a satisfying and fulfilling purpose – is to introduce this inner child to a *neutrality of will*. This is a very simple idea. It basically means being willing to consider lots of different options, without getting all wrapped up in any particular one. If we can gently hold everything within and without at arms length – all the knowledge, emotions, experiences, plans, insights, relationships and nourishment – without committing to any particular course of action, we begin to cultivate a neutrality of will. It's like caring about someone, but letting them find their own way without trying to control them. Or allowing the circumstances of our life to unfold around us without being forceful, controlling or needy.

The reason this is important is that if we become too attached to either what we desire or what happens around us – if we are always yearning and striving and pining – then this restricts our will from taking shape in the world, and restricts our purpose from fulfilling itself. Instead, we must learn how to be engaged but neutral. Imagine that you have been given a magic ball that you can throw as far as you want – even to the moon! But if you are always holding onto that ball, desperately clinging to it out of fear and worry, it will never go anywhere. And the same is true of our will and purpose. If we clutch them too tightly or try to control them too completely, they will not have the freedom to find the most fulfilling ways to be expressed. So we must cradle our dreams and visions loosely, like a tiny feather that could blow out of our hands at any moment.

How can we help Pemba understand what *neutrality of will* looks and feels like? Well, interestingly, if we take good care of all our other inner children, they will all be learning how to be engaged but neutral in their own self-nurturing. Wachiwi will have more physical strength, energy and flexibility because she is free to dance. Manjit will be smarter, faster and more agile because he has learned how to watch himself from a place of stillness. Adelyte will have more emotional depth and range because we encourage her to be playful and free in her creative expressions. Shen will have access to more insight and wisdom when we encourage him to softly touch our inner Light without grasping after it greedily. In each of these cases, we are encouraging each child to be neutral but engaged, caring but carefree, active but not compulsive, compassionate but not clingy. In practicing all of these together, we help Pemba learn to let go while being inspired and courageous at the same time.

As already discussed, Pemba also needs to have some way of knowing whether we are actually fulfilling our life's purpose or not – some way of measuring our progress. So before you go to bed at night, write down a few questions about what you are doing the next day, considering how they will affect your chosen purpose. For instance: "Is the educational or career path I am taking really helping me fulfill my purpose, or is it interfering with it?" or "Are the friendships or romantic relationships I am in supporting the purpose of my life, or distracting me from it?" or "Does the recreation I am about to engage in align with the vision I have for my life, or not?" or "Are tomorrow's activities an expression of who I sincerely and authentically am?" And so on...whatever makes the most sense for what you plan to be doing that day. Then, when you wake up in the morning, ask yourself those same questions before you do anything else – before you have started your daily routine or even fully woken up – and keep track of the feelings and sensations that arise inside you in response to each question. This will help Pemba evaluate whether we are on track with our life's purpose or not.

There are other steps we can take to allow our will to flourish and our purpose to become fully real in our lives. And Pemba already knows how to lead us there. We just need to let Pemba know that we think our purpose is important – as important as any other nourishment for any other inner child. And we need to be patient and persistent, because the meaning and purpose of our life may take years to fully unfold for us. But if we care for Pemba, Pemba will care for us. Love is a reciprocal exchange that amplifies itself – this is one of the miracles of all relationships. And the more sincerely, freely and skillfully we offer our love, the more every inner child can help us find our way to a fulfilling and self-empowered life. So we give, we lavish with affection and kindness, and then we let go, knowing that whatever we have loved in this way will flourish and endure.

Questions for Reflection & Discussion

- What has your relationship with Pemba been like? Do you feel you have a sense of purpose? Why or why not?

- Do you think all of your inner children can work in harmony toward a common purpose? Why or why not?

- Have you observed other people with a strong sense of purpose? What are some of the signs that this is so?

- Have you ever experienced someone else's sense of purpose influencing you or "taking over" your own plans?

- How does your Pemba's sense of purpose differ from your Fabian's concerns about a legacy? How are they similar?

- Have you ever experienced a *neutrality of will* in some situation? If so, what did it feel like for you?

- Why do you think it might be unhealthy or unwise to ignore our own sense of purpose for too long?

- What is the most nurturing thing you could do for Pemba in the next twenty-four hours?

HARMONIZING TWELVE DIMENSIONS

All this time we have been using the metaphor of inner children to describe each of the twelve dimensions of self. Really we could interact with these dimensions in any number of ways, but envisioning them as unique individuals with their own personalities, wants and needs helps us understand how a loving relationship with every aspect of self is the key to being well and whole. There is one more step in creating truly balanced and harmonious nourishment, and that is combining our perceptions, understanding and practices in ways that create a whole that is greater than the sum of its parts. This is the "integral" part of Integral Lifework. For even though it is a wonderful thing to ensure our inner family is cared for individually, to be fully nourished we must celebrate the unity of our whole self. Our whole self is a mixture of all its parts – a synthesis that is more creative, more alive, more ingenious and more powerful than any one aspect of our being by itself. And one of the simplest ways we can recognize and energize this unity of our total being is to maintain regular forms of *integral practice* – that is, habits that create harmonious nourishment between all of our inner children at once.

Integral practice can be developed in a number of ways. One of them is unconscious and spontaneous. For example, as you continue to work through the exercises in each chapter that help you connect with each inner child, something miraculous begins to occur. Without even realizing it, you will combine these techniques into a daily routine that naturally includes different dimensions. One way this happens is that, after practicing these exercises for a while, elements of each exercise will find their way into our regular patterns of being. For example, we might find ourselves slipping into the Watcher perspective during the day to observe what Manjit is up to. Or we might hear Nobuko's voice more often and clearly as she examines the integrity of our thoughts, feelings, words and actions in each moment. Or we may find Luceria helping us switch from one mode of interaction to another more fluidly, without our even thinking about it. And so on. All of this can happen without our actively trying or thinking about it.

Another way that integral practices develop is when a particular exercise or routine taps into many different dimensions at once, nourishing many or even all of our inner kids at the same time. We could call this a "layered" activity. For example, an exercise that focuses on Shen might nurture Wachiwi and Pemba at the same time. Or a conversation with Irina may provide nourishment to Adelyte and Asim. Everything within us is so interconnected, almost any practice can become layered, and we won't necessarily realize all the different ways we are being nourished until much later. Sometimes we may choose to consciously develop activities that combine several nourishing routines into a layered routine. I have designed many such layered activities over time, and, by experimenting with different combinations, have found one or two that work well for me for a few years. But each of us must experiment on our own to synthesize layered activities uniquely suited to who we are. And what works for a few months or years may require changes and adjustments to remain useful. There is no one-size-fits-all approach, and it is important to add variety and surprises so our inner kids don't get bored.

One of the most powerful integral tools of all is just to be aware, as frequently and attentively as possible, that all of those inner children require our loving relationship. They all want to be remembered, so they can participate in everything we do. So when we are working hard at a job or in school, or when we spend time doing something fun, or when we are laboring through chores at home, or when we take a trip somewhere exciting and new, in each situation or environment we can find ways to include all of our inner kids. Let's say we are going to the store or market to obtain something we need. Wachiwi will be overjoyed if we walk or ride a bicycle there, so she has a chance to be nourished.

Manjit will delight in looking at different things – even things we aren't interested in acquiring – to learn something new about the world. Eilon will be thrilled if we talk to different people around us and create new connections and relationships. Pemba will be delighted if we can figure out how today's learning and interactions contribute to our life's purpose. Adelyte will take joy in observing the market through a creative lens of some kind – making sketches, taking pictures, recording sounds or writing down observations. Nobuko will be content if we follow through on something we promised ourselves or someone else we would do at the market. And so on. The more we can bring to mind all of our inner kids as we go about our daily routines, the more they will excitedly participate in our day-to-day life in a layered and integral way.

All of this will unfold differently for everyone – there is no set formula for how a person's integral practice evolves. It will also continue to evolve over time. Of course we may need to work through any barriers we come across during our journey – that is, we may need to target certain dimensions of self that don't receive a lot of regular nourishment, and try to better understand why we might be avoiding or neglecting them. We may even want to carefully construct a "Lifework Plan," which will help us keep track of where we are, where we want to go, and any areas of special focus or effort we want to include. Keeping some sort of journal for each of our nourishment dimensions and the benefits we experience with different nourishment routines can be extremely helpful over time. Yet regardless of how we proceed, it is always important to continue listening to our inner children, and to be willing to change course on a moment's notice. As we discover how nurturing occurs for us – in this moment, across all dimensions – we should always feel free to flow in new directions according to those inner promptings and discoveries.

It goes without saying that all of our efforts must continue to be guided by the right intention, too. The golden intention – desiring the good of All above anything else – is a powerful ally in caring for every dimension of self. For when we hold the golden intention in our heart, we begin to expand our compassion into larger and larger circles of caring. At first we are lavishing compassionate kindness on our inner kids, and once they feel strong and safe, our compassion will overflow into our closest relationships. Those relationships then benefit from the

same multidimensional nourishment that our inner children do. Our
Wachiwi begins to encourage the Wachiwi in others, and receives
encouragement in return. Our Shen connects with the Shen in others.
Our Adelyte celebrates with the Adelyte in others. Our Pemba discovers
ways to support the Pemba in others, and in turn be supported by them.
We may not connect with everyone the same way, but if the good of All
guides our interactions, natural harmonies will grow from a foundation
of mutual respect, appreciation and love.

Eventually, as we maintain the golden intention, this expansion of love
and nurturing through integral practice will continue into all the realms
of our life. Into our school and workplace, our surrounding community,
the city we live in or near, and ever outward. It will influence what we
buy and where we shop. It will change how we view and participate in
politics and government. It will lead us into new and powerful ways of
nourishing our region, our nation and humanity as a whole. It will
nudge us into greater harmony with the natural systems of the Earth, so
that these too are nourished in every dimension. And even beyond the
Earth – into our solar system, our galaxy and farther still – our
compassionate intention will find mysterious and inexplicable ways to
express itself wisely and skillfully. If we keep grounding ourselves in a
desire for the greatest good, for the most all-encompassing effect
possible, our circles of love and caring will continually expand to
embrace the Universe itself.

Integral Harmony, Integral Symphony

As we create more and more integral activities where every aspect of self
is being nourished in some way – and then, slowly but inevitably, every
aspect of other people and the world around us is being nurtured as well
– something truly magical happens. The wholeness and wellness that
we generate begins to amplify itself. What starts as each dimension of
our being learning how to individually thrive and sing eventually
becomes a chorus of joyful and energetic voices. And the harmonious
music of that chorus is contagious. There is no way to contain it.
Because it is grounded in love and affection, everyone and everything it
touches will want to become part of the music. And the more people
who join in song – the more voices that harmonize with the principles of

integral nourishment – the louder and more resonant the music becomes. Eventually, a great symphony of Love, Life, Liberty and Light arises spontaneously out of this harmony, reaching across vast distances to celebrate every aspect of existence. It is a symphony that takes the tiniest gestures of kindness and echoes them among the furthest galaxies. Perhaps this symphony is already playing within us and around us all of the time, and we are just learning to tune into it and sing along. Or perhaps we are the very instruments that bring that symphony into being. Who knows what is really at work here? But to whatever degree we develop and sustain integral practice, we will begin to glimpse the magnificent choreography of the Universe, and hear the soaring melodies of every interconnected thing within and without.

HEALING SAD, ANGRY OR REBELLIOUS KIDS

Have you ever met someone who doesn't seem very happy? Unhappiness can take many forms, so sometimes it's hard to recognize at first. Maybe they act withdrawn and quiet most of the time, and whenever anyone tries to talk to them, they avoid that person or become embarrassed. Maybe they even push someone away when that person tries to make friends with them. But a sad person may also be someone who gets angry easily, starts arguments all the time, seems to always get in trouble with authority, or finds other ways of demanding attention all the time. For these people, being sad means they are boisterous and pushy instead of quiet and shy. Sad people can also be people who are always looking out for others, always putting themselves in risky situations to defend someone or make someone else feel better. For this last group of people, as strange as it seems, taking risks to help others while depriving themselves is how they show their sadness.

So we could say that there are three types of sad people: people who see themselves as victims (the quiet, shy types); people who see themselves as abusers (the loud, demanding, bullying types); and people who see themselves as rescuers (always helping others, often at risk to their own well-being). Why does sadness look so different in different people? Sometimes this has to do with a person's natural personality. But it is also because people tend to treat others the way they themselves have been treated, or because they are imitating the examples of people who have been closest to them throughout their life. So someone who sees one parent angrily yelling at the other parent might become an abuser themselves, or they might feel more like a victim and act that way instead, or they might become the rescuer in the family, defending other family members when an abusive parent goes on a rampage. And so what is really happening here is that people are learning to cope with their pain and sadness by becoming the very sort of person that made them feel hurt and sad in the first place. Because of this process of observation and imitation, even naturally shy and sensitive people can sometimes become bullies, naturally angry and aggressive people can become rescuers, and naturally helpful people can become victims.

What is even stranger is that when you put a sad person in a different situation with different sorts of pressures and challenges, they may take on any of these three roles. An abuser might become a victim, a victim might become a rescuer, a rescuer an abuser, and so on. For example, let's say I'm eight years old and resentful of my six-year-old sister because she ate all of my favorite snack food and got away with it, and now she's even teasing me about it. I feel like a victim and see her as an abuser. So to "get even," I steal her favorite shirt and hide it underneath my bed. When my sister discovers her shirt is gone, she feels like a victim and becomes very upset. My sister then runs crying to our mom, who becomes a rescuer by consoling my sister and telling her everything will be all right. Our mom then comes into my room, finds the shirt, and punishes me with loud yelling and threats of further punishment. As she is yelling, I begin to cry and wail, feeling like a victim all over again. My sister, who at first was feeling pretty smug and righteous, now feels sorry for me and intervenes like a rescuer – she begs our mom not to be so angry and not to punish me further. Then mom gets angry at my sister for interfering, and so on…. So over the course of one day, a sad person can change roles many times, just trying to cope with the stress and pain they are feeling, and thereby participate in all sorts of drama. When you gather a whole group of sad people together, they can end up acting out these roles towards each other constantly! And when such people hurt really badly inside, they often believe they can't react any other way.

What is so unfortunate about this situation is that none of these roles will help sad people feel any better, resolve any of the problems they face, or help them be better nourished. In fact, if they can't free themselves from this cycle of acting out victim-rescuer-abuser roles, they will just feel worse and worse over time. Sadness just makes more sadness. So the victim becomes more and more withdrawn, depriving themselves of more and more nourishment. The abuser becomes more and more demanding, trying harder and harder to dominate and control everyone and everything around them. The rescuer becomes more and more desperate to help others, at greater expense to their own well-being. And all of this begins when a person isn't being loved in ways that nurture and support them; when one or more of their inner children is being gravely undernourished.

And how do our inner kids respond to this? Whenever a member of our inner family isn't being nourished with kindness and care, they too adopt rescuer, abuser or victim roles. Imagine what it would be like if your Lada was frequently scolded or humiliated and never allowed to be cared for at all? Or what if your Pemba was never given an opportunity to find his purpose? What if your Shen was laughed at and ridiculed, or your Adelyte was never allowed to creatively express herself? What if your Wachiwi was purposely hurt over and over again? Whenever our inner children are restricted, abused or starved in such ways, they can't help but adopt victim, abuser and rescuer roles and unconsciously continue that deprivation. As victims, they give up trying to be nourished, or don't believe they deserve to be cared for at all, and push away our efforts to love them. As rescuers, they focus all of their energy on their fellow siblings while neglecting their own needs, and become more and more depleted over time. As abusers, they act out or try to take over, demanding more nourishment and attention at the expense of their brothers and sisters. And, what is worse, once our inner kids have started down this path, they begin to believe that these are the only choices available to them.

Even as we start becoming aware of particular inner family members that are rebellious, underdeveloped or uncared for, our own first instinct as a parent may be to rescue them, to see them as victims. Or perhaps we will become angry and try to control them or force them to improve, as any abuser would. Or maybe we will just give in and give up, because that's what a victim is supposed to do. Even as the parent who should know better, we often can't help but act out the abuser-victim-rescuer roles over and over again. Until we learn a new way of being, our inner kids will continue to deprive themselves, and as their parent we will continue to contribute to the self-depleting drama. In order to heal and grow, we need to learn new ways of engaging our sad, rebellious kids. We need to learn something we may never have observed or experienced before. Somehow, we need to teach them as gently as possible how to start caring for themselves after years of neglect. We need to learn to love them in the most healthy, joyful and supportive ways possible.

The Conversation

In order to relearn how to nurture our neglected inner kids – and to listen to them with love – we almost always need to have those skills modeled by someone else. Remember that this is how we learn to be a rescuer, abuser or victim in the first place: by the examples we observe. It is probably not possible to learn a new way of being just from reading or attending a class or lecture. This particular healing process usually requires the assistance of someone who understands the barriers we are facing and how to help us overcome them. In essence, we need a "moderator" for our dialogue with our inner family – a sort of referee who can show us how to listen and respond with skilled and loving kindness. Often this is someone who has overcome adversity themselves, who has had to let go of the abuser-victim-rescuer cycle in their own life. There have been many people over the years who helped me tremendously in this way. These ranged from school teachers to social workers to foster parents to family therapists to spiritual counselors to close personal friends. I count myself as blessed to have encountered so many healing influences, and it was because of them that I was inspired to be a healing presence for others. And we can find these sorts of people everywhere *if we allow it to happen*. If we permit ourselves to become vulnerable, to ask for help when we need it, to seek out people who are skilled and compassionate listeners, they will begin to show up in our lives.

Do these have to be professionals? Not necessarily, because it is quite difficult to obtain a degree or certificate in empathy, compassion and intuition – and these are the talents most required. At the same time, those people who are drawn to certain professions often tend to have these innate abilities. Even so, we will still need to be discerning in whom we choose to ask for help, because not everyone who is a teacher can teach well, not everyone who is a spiritual counselor can counsel wisely, not everyone who is a social worker has empathy, not everyone who is a therapist is a good listener, and not all of our close friends have accurate intuition. Still, if we are blind in some area (such as being discerning), how can we rely on ourselves to find the right people to help us see? This is very difficult, and often requires a number of baby steps to get from the place where we first acknowledge we need help to a place where we actually obtain that help.

The first baby step is to recognize our own needs, where we can say to ourselves, "Hey, I'm not very good at this self-nourishment stuff!" It isn't enough to just be upset about failing in some way, we also need to recognize that we are at least partly responsible for wherever we are – and completely responsible for finding a new direction. The second baby step is opening ourselves up to receiving help with our journey – to let someone else into our process and trust them to hold our hand for a while. At the same time, we shouldn't rely on anyone to always be there for us – we would never learn how to walk on our own if we did that – but we have to be willing to lean on others if we keep stumbling and falling in some area. The third baby step is to try really hard to listen to what that trusted resource shares with us, and to be willing to try out some of the things they suggest we do. It is often easier to ask for help than it is to accept and integrate that help once it is offered. Why? Because we may need to change how we think about ourselves, or about others, or about a particular situation...and accepting that we need to change can be hard.

Whoever we allow to help us with our process may offer us many different approaches to change how we think about ourselves. There is, however, one kind of approach that I have found more helpful than any other in working with my own healing, and when helping others heal. The essence of this approach is listening to our inner dialogues, replaying our earliest memories, and observing our feelings from moment-to-moment to understand what patterns exist there. Are there lots of images, words and feelings that convince us we can't nourish ourselves in some way? Do particular memories, phrases or emotions replay themselves over and over again, somehow paralyzing or sabotaging us? If so, are those patterns really necessary or justifiable?

Are they grounded in what is happening right now, or stuck in some past experience? Do they reflect what is real, or just what is imagined?

For example, what if I always told myself "You are a terrible dancer!" every time someone asked me to dance? Or what if I always felt ashamed or anxious every time I took a bath, without knowing why? Or what if the strongest memories from my childhood – ones that always seem easily brought to mind – are about someone being cruel to me when I was little? An approach that works well with these patterns is simply to challenge them. To say "Hey, wait a minute! Am I really a bad dancer? Or did someone just tell me I was once?" or "What is so bad about sitting in a tub of hot water? Am I afraid I'm going to drown? What is making me feel this way...?" or "What does this memory of a cruel person have to do with who I am today? Is the situation I was in then still valid in the present? Are there other ways I can view what happened to me back then that free me to be different today?" In many ways, we are revisiting the inner realms that Irina, Asim and Adelyte control. But we are doing it in a very structured and disciplined way, and having a very specific kind of conversation with them. We are examining those realms with special care, and testing the patterns we see there. We are asking why those patterns exist at all, and how we might want to change them. So, if you can, try to find someone who can help you use this kind of approach.

It is important to remember that all of these baby steps can take time to achieve. So, just as with so much else in life, patience, self-discipline and the courage to follow-through will part of the deal as well. And we must always remember that it is incredibly easy to revert back into acting like a victim, abuser or rescuer throughout this process. Those old roles may feel safe and familiar, and shaking them off will take lots of practice. So the fourth baby step is really just sticking to it. To steadfastly endure and keep taking the first three steps over and over again until we begin to see positive changes; to continue believing change is possible until that change occurs. It doesn't really matter how we maintain this belief, as long as we can *keep believing.* Maybe we'll start from a place of tenderness and hurt, and rely on that feeling as a reason to keep trudging along. Maybe we'll get angry along the way, and let that anger fuel our efforts for a time. Maybe we'll discover that we can forgive ourselves or someone else for something that happened to us, and ride that wave of forgiveness into our next phase of inner work. Maybe we'll experience some success in our healing process, and rely on the joy of that victory to encourage ourselves to keep moving forward. However we can find it, we must have faith that we can heal and grow and change, and that we must do these things for the good of All. Sometimes this requires willpower and determination, sometimes it requires letting go, and sometimes it requires both. But we experience the tiniest bit of faith and allow that faith to help feed and heal our inner kids, our inner family will be strengthened through that effort, and will then begin to work in concert to help us continue that nourishment and healing.

How to Care When We Don't

There is one final challenge to our inner parenting, and that is how to remain motivated and energized with loving kindness over time. In a way, the simple act of remembering each of our inner kids, of spending just a little time with them each day, is one way to keep the flame of love burning bright within our inner family. A child's natural inclination when we care for them is to thrive and grow; they love attention and encouragement, they blossom from being understood and appreciated, and that may be enough in itself. In other words, when we nourish every member of our inner family, we will experience an upwelling of compassion and affection as a natural consequence. Our inner kids will lavish affection on us, and we will feel content and whole, which in turn will help us continue to have energy enough to care for all of them. In the natural sciences, they call this a positive feedback loop – energy that naturally amplifies itself. This creates a natural harmony and momentum that keeps us moving forward.

In this way we have a built-in mechanism for maintaining our success. Once we have begun regularly listening to our inner children – once we have demonstrated to them that we really care – they will regularly remind us of what they need. Wachiwi will let us know that she is getting antsy and wants to play. Manjit will pester us with curiosity about some new topic of interest. Shen will continually nudge us into deeper connection with our ground of being. Adelyte will keep pulling our attention away from whatever we are doing into a daydream of creative activity she wants to pursue. Irina will remind us of memories that we need to explore and organize. Pemba will create situations where our purpose can be fulfilled if we are willing to seize the day and follow through.   Eilon will prod us into new connections and relationships with others. Luceria will insist we provide equal time for all of our interior modes of interaction. And so on. The clamor and prompting from our inner children will be constant. In a way, once we establish healthy, nurturing relationships with our inner family, it is nearly impossible to avoid healing, growth and transformation, because the pattern for that progress has become clear. When all of our inner children have experienced what it looks and feels like to be whole, they won't want to turn back.

There are exceptions, however; there will be times when this natural momentum is interrupted. Especially during times of stress, or when we feel overwhelmed and can't make time to care for all our inner kids, or when we are depressed for some reason we haven't yet understood, it may be hard to care at all. What can we do in these situations? In the last chapter, we saw how patterns and roles from our childhood may keep us from being able to nourish our inner family, so the first thing we will want to do is examine ourselves for any evidence of this kind of self-sabotage. Are we acting out victim, abuser or rescuer roles? We can also check in with others who know us well to see if they have observed any such tendencies. We might want to join one of the Coregroups described in the next chapter to see how others are coping, seek emotional support for our journey, and just relax into the flow of that community. And of course we can also seek the opinion of a professional therapist or counselor to gain an independent perspective. However, if we exhaust all of these measures and still can't reinvigorate our passion for caring, then we will need to come at things from another angle. We will need to discover new ways to find joy and compassion, even when the hope of authentic caring seems like a distant possibility.

For example, as a starting point, here are some questions you can ask yourself when positive motivations seem hard to come by:

- **"What do I want more than anything else?"** What is it you yearn for? What is missing in your life? What end result do you cherish in your heart? What picture is in our mind that you want to become real?   What options or possibilities cry out to you?

- **"What do I believe would make my life better?"**   What conditions do you feel need to occur for you to be more content? What event or change do you think would help you be more at peace with yourself and your environment?   What could happen today that would make tomorrow feel like a brighter day?

- **"What is most important to me?"**   What do you value more than anything else?   What do you hold most dear in your heart? What sorts of events in the world make you sit up and take notice?   What do you find yourself thinking about most of the time?   What inspires the strongest (positive or negative) emotional reactions in you?

Spending some time delving into these questions can, by itself, lead us to surprising places, because they nudge us into better awareness about our desires, goals and priorities – whatever those may be. If you are feeling a bit paralyzed or out-of-balance, I would encourage you to take time to think about these questions. For we all have desires, goals and priorities, whether we realize it or not…they are there, floating beneath the surface of our thoughts, waiting for us to reach down and pull them up for a closer look. Sometimes talking to someone else – a close friend, a family member, or a professional therapist – will help us explore these questions. Sometimes writing our thoughts down in a personal journal will help us identify and keep track of our desires, goals and priorities. Sometimes meditating in silence on the questions above for a few minutes each day will encourage fully formed answers to rise up out of the velvety dark within over time. Whatever approach you think will help you most, please give it a try.

Now, once we begin to better understand our desires, goals and priorities, we can explore things further with more questions. Perhaps the most important one, and the one we will need to ask over and over again, is *"Why?"* Why do we want what we want? Why do we believe something will make us happier? Why do we think a certain thing is important? Understanding the "whys" leads us deeper into ourselves, to the places inside where the raw materials behind all of our wants, beliefs and assumptions reside. Those raw materials are very powerful; they are a kind of magic that lives deep down in every human being. And as we come to understand the "whys" more clearly and completely, we set that magic loose.

And here's the really interesting thing about this process: sometimes, when we begin asking these kinds of questions, we discover that the answers don't really line up with each other very well. That is, the answers to a few or even all of these questions somehow contradict each other, or don't really make much sense. If my answers to the questions "What do I believe would make life better?" and "What do I want more than anything else?" and "What is most important to me?" are all different, then that means I am being pulled in many different directions at once. If this is the case, then it won't be that surprising if I am unhappy, or feel stuck and unable to move forward, or have stopped caring very much. Looking carefully at how honest answers to each of these questions line up with each other will open our eyes to any competing feelings or beliefs we may have. Then, when we ask "why" about each one of those feelings or beliefs, we can dig down even further to a common ground beneath them all. For common ground is there, if we dig deep enough. Remember that this will take time, patience and the courage to persist. At first, it really doesn't matter if we care about this process, just that we keep trying it until some answers begin to emerge.

Now what do I mean by "common ground?" In once sense, I mean what drives everything we do. But I also mean something more. For even though each of us will experience them differently, we all share fundamental drives that inspire all human wants and needs. For example, on some level we are driven to exist; we are driven to remain alive and remain aware of being alive. We are also driven to experience the world around us in various ways – to see, touch, taste, hear and feel that world. And we are driven to adapt – to learn the best, most effective ways of interacting with that world – so that we can continue to exist and fully experience life. And finally we are also driven to affect what happens to us and to our environment; we want to cause changes that demonstrate clearly and loudly to ourselves and others that we are existing, experiencing and learning. These four fundamental drives – to exist, experience, adapt and affect – are the enduring foundation for all of our desires, goals and priorities. They are the bedrock upon which our reasons for living, thinking, feeling, and choosing a course of action are built. And when we delve down deeply into ourselves, asking questions about our own priorities, wants, hopes and *whys*, we will begin to connect with our fundamental drives. Once again, these may express themselves quite differently for each person. But if we avoid seeking out this fundamental connection, we risk living in a tense battle with the very energies that give us life.

Once you have uncovered the common ground of your desires, goals and priorities, you are ready for the next step. Here are a few more questions to help you on your way:

- **"What will happen to me?"** How will what you think is important, or what you want, or what you think makes life better affect you? How will you be changed? What will your personal world look like?

- **"What can I do to help?"** How can you assist in making what you want, what you think is important, and what you believe would make life better a lasting reality? What sorts of things can you do to make that happen?

- **"What is the very next step I can take to move forward?"** What single thing can you do to set things in motion? What can you say or do that will nudge conditions from where they are right now to what you believe is most important, what will make life better, and what you truly most desire?

These are the additional questions we should keep asking over and over, even as things begin to change as a result of our efforts. And of course we need to be realistic about all of this. As with all journeys we undertake, we must exercise patience, not take too much on at once, and occasionally check in with our answers to the first set of questions again – just to see if we are still on track. Are we really moving forward? Are we getting closer to our goals? And of course our answers to all of these questions should continue to align with each other, working together harmoniously rather than in opposition. And as we slowly move in the direction of what we value most, we will begin to become more invested in our day-to-day self-nourishing practices. We will begin to commit our heart to the outcomes we envision. We will begin to care.

At this point, if we continue to explore these self-inquiry exercises, our motivations to nurture our inner children will likely change and evolve, but they will always remain positive and supportive. In fact, for most of us, taking care of our inner family will become the first and foremost "next step" each day. Why? Because what becomes clear over time is that, when we renew and refresh our motivation, we renew and refresh all kinds of nourishment for our inner kids. And as we support that inner family, we will discover new and surprising reasons each day to live, thrive and chart our course through life.

Are there other special recipes for overcoming indifference in some area, or inspiring greater willpower to move forward? Is there some ultimate secret to being able to care more? Yes, there is, and we have already touched upon it in previous chapters. The golden intention is the key to energized and enduring kindness, compassion and caring. For the more we perfect an inclusive love for everything and everyone, the more we are driven to nourish and sustain what is good for everyone and everything – including ourselves. And as we persevere in our efforts, our understanding of what the "good of All" really is will also continue to evolve. We will refine our understanding of compassionate affection and become more and more skilled and wise in its application. We will tend to let go of our old modes of being and embrace new ones. We will transform ourselves and the world around us in unexpected ways. And, although the "whys" of our efforts will still remain – and may even become more transparent and obvious as we continue along our path – having such detailed explanations will become less important. Even when we face doubts, disruptions and failures, we will always have the means to find our way, and the energy and endurance to renew our compassion. How? Because we have built our integral practice around the needs and voices of our inner family, and we will always have their steadfast help to guide and inspire our journey.

OUR PARTNERS IN PARENTING

Before we come to the end of this book, I think it is important that we not feel alone in these efforts to take care of our inner family, or to heal and grow in any dimension of self. This should not be viewed as a solitary effort, and in fact trying to do it all by ourselves can add a lot of unnecessary stress to the journey. As we've already discussed in previous chapters, in some instances it may not even be possible to be a good parent without help. So the following are some invaluable resources for anyone who wants to begin the inspiring adventure of self-nourishment and sustain it over time.

Integral Coregroups

As our Eilon is likely to remind us, as social beings we need other people, and other people need us. We shouldn't put unnecessary pressure on ourselves and try to "go it alone." What at first may seem simpler or less complicated when we don't involve others quickly becomes stressful and overwhelming without a community of support. In this sense, parenting our inner children is just like real parenting, where sometimes we just need other parents to talk to about what we are going through and how we might approach particular challenges. There is also a something special that happens when people get together – a kind of deep sharing and inner learning that may not happen at all when we are alone. Having some sort of regular get-together with a diverse group of people to work on Integral Lifework issues is an essential part of growth, healing and transformation.   And that is what Integral Coregroups are meant to provide.

The basic idea of how these groups work has come from many years of teaching classes, leading discussions, and being involved with support groups of many different types.   And although the idea is simple, it won't always come naturally, and may take some practice.   What makes this approach so different is that it asks participants to follow a specific format, and provides guidelines of how to interact with each other in a group.   The format and guidelines call upon us to be humble, compassionate and self-controlled in ways that may seem uncomfortable at first, but which really pay off in the long run in extraordinary ways.

The format of the group is a combination of guided discussion and meditation. The "Guide" can be anyone, and in fact I encourage that role to rotate among all members of the group, with a new Guide for each session.   If it's a newly established group, anyone can be a Guide.   With an established group, participants should attend at least four sessions before volunteering for the role of Guide.   The Guide's responsibility is to offer up the discussion questions, allow everyone in the group to participate, to remind people of guidelines if they forget them, and to follow the format below as closely as possible.   The Guide doesn't answer the questions or comment on them, but encourages everyone else to do so and keeps the discussion going.   The ideal Integral Coregroup size is between six and twelve people, and the format of each session goes like this:

- Everyone is given time to find a seat, take some refreshment if that is offered, and visit a little with each other. This might be for ten minutes or so.

- The Guide then invites people to "check in."   This gives everyone an opportunity to share their name (just their first name or however they would like to be addressed), what is going on in their lives right now, any brief announcements they would like to make about upcoming events or resources they think the group would be interested in, and why they have come to this particular session.   The check-in should take another fifteen minutes or so.

- The Guide then introduces the topic for the session – which all of the questions will relate to in some way – and then briefly covers the guidelines for participation (outlined below), including the 90-minute time limit.

- The Guide then starts the session by inviting everyone to take a moment of silence together to set their intention for the following hour. That intention is an inner commitment to "the good of All," however each person feels this in their heart. This is sort of a prayer or meditation that projects goodwill and loving kindness from each person in the group towards everyone else in the group. This might just be a feeling of goodwill and love, or it might be words spoken silently that set our intention. An example of this would be: "May Love and Light arise in me today, and in everyone else here, so that whatever is healing, strengthening and nourishing can radiate through each of us into the world at large."

- After a minute or two, the Guide indicates that the discussion is beginning. The Guide then asks the first question and leads the group in a minute or two of silent introspection in response to the question. The Guide then invites people to share whatever answers (or additional questions) they have found within themselves. Every person who guides will have a different style of encouraging this sharing. Perhaps they will offer additional questions about each question that is asked. But whatever they do, they must walk a fine line between inviting and encouraging discussion, and pressuring people who aren't ready to participate. In a well-established group of people who already know each other, discussion will likely unfold naturally and easily. In a new group, some people may understandably be hesitant or shy.

- Whenever someone responds to a question, the Guide will thank them for their thoughts – without judging or evaluating what they have said – and then ask other people to add their own contributions. If someone is taking much more time than others in the group, or interrupting others, or for some reason isn't able to follow the guidelines below, then it is the Guide's responsibility to gently and compassionately help them understand this. Hopefully, though, the Guide's main focus can be to create an inviting space for everyone to contribute. The Guide does not contribute any answers to the questions while they are guiding.

- If participants do have questions about the topic or the questions being asked, the Guide will redirect them to the rest of the group for answers. The Guide is not an authority here – in fact there are no authorities. There are only hearts, minds and souls seeking within themselves for answers. If someone has need of specific resources (introductory materials on the concepts of Integral Lifework, the services of an Integral Lifework practitioner, other resources, etc.), the more established or well-versed members of the group may encourage them to seek those resources outside of the group, but Integral Coregroups are not intended to be a marketing or networking opportunity for professional services.

- When the session reaches the 90-minute mark, the Guide then reminds people of the time limit, thanks everyone for their participation, and then wraps up the topical discussion for that session. At this point, anyone who wants to stay to discuss business items can stay, and anyone who wants to leave can leave. This is a good time to have a ten minute break before beginning the business portion of the session.

- After everyone has settled back down, the Guide reminds people of any old business that needs to be addressed, of new business that needs to be decided upon, and invites people to bring up any new business items. This part of the session is often about logistics – who will Guide the next session, where to meet, what time the session will occur, who might need help with transportation, etc. It also might include discussion about social get-togethers, like potlucks, walks in Nature or other group activities. This part of the session should take no more than a half hour, so that the total Integral Coregroup session does not exceed two-and-a-half hours. Some simplified version of

"Robert's Rules of Order" can be helpful for the business portion
of the meeting, but groups can come up with their own way of
doing business – whatever works!

You can see how the Guide has a lot of responsibility for helping the
session be supportive and enriching. People with different personalities
and strengths will have different approaches to guiding, but the intent is
always the same: to empower the participants. Of course, the Guide
isn't alone in this. Each participant should also commit to helping each
session be as successful as possible by following guidelines below.
Because everyone will have the opportunity to become Guides
themselves, that will help the group members build skills to support
each other.

So here are the guidelines for participation, which are the foundation of
the Integral Coregroup itself, and in many ways more important than the
Guide's role:

- **Avoiding crosstalk.** Participants may be inspired to share
  something in response to something another member says.
  However, there are no right or wrong answers to most
  questions. There is also no need to correct someone else's
  misunderstanding…unless they themselves ask for clarification.
  Thus all answers and questions should be directed to the group
  as a whole, not specific people, and participants should refrain
  from reacting to what someone else shares – other than perhaps
  echoing the Guide's appreciation and thanks for that sharing.
  For example, I might say "I appreciate what s/he just said,
  because it resonates strongly with something I also feel…"
  Participants should be very careful not to speak directly to other
  members of the group during the session, but speak to everyone
  as a group. Each person should feel safe and supported in
  sharing whatever they like, as long as that sharing follows the
  other guidelines below.

- **Appreciating diversity.** Participants are to be as accepting as
  possible of all types of people, and all points of view, within the
  Integral Coregroup session. If everyone thought and felt exactly
  the same way about everything, these groups would not be very

enriching...or very interesting! Even when someone says something we think is appalling or offensive, we must train our heart to be compassionate and understanding, rather than judgmental or hostile. We might offer an alternate point of view to the group, but we must recognize that whenever this starts a back-and-forth between two or more participants, things can quickly turn into a debate. And that is not what Integral Coregroups are about. They are about sharing from our heart, then letting go. About listening from the heart, and letting that go, too. If we are in doubt about how to process what someone has shared, we should take a moment to close our eyes, breathe deeply and see past their words into the heart of the person speaking them. After all, that heart is just like ours, with all its pain, grief and joy.

- **Nonviolent speech.** The idea that things we say can hurt each other is not a revolutionary idea. But to create a safe and inviting place for people to share themselves openly, we must be especially careful with the words we use. Speech that expresses prejudice, hatred or disdain is not helpful. Speech that makes us right and someone else wrong is not helpful – especially because the real truth usually lies somewhere in the middle anyway. Words that belittle or embarrass others do not encourage openness. We may have feelings of anger over something being discussed, but in this group, such feelings should never translate into yelling at someone, or calling them nasty names, or putting someone down because they believe or think a certain way. Whenever we feel a strong reaction rising up that we can't control, and that we suspect will disrupt the harmony of the group, we should excuse ourselves from the group for a few minutes to be alone and regain our composure, then return when we are ready.

- **Compassionate silence.** Sometimes a certain topic or question may uncover a well of painful memories and emotions in one or more members of the group. But participants should commit to letting that pain be expressed without trying to comfort or rescue the person in pain. And when I am the person feeling pain – even if I am crying my heart out – I should also not expect other participants to comfort me or change my emotional state. I should not expect anyone to reach out to me, or try to make me feel better. Practicing "compassionate silence" means that the group accepts the pain of one person and allows it to just be. No actions need to be taken. No one needs to respond at all, other than the Guide who will express gratitude for the sharing, and perhaps create some extra time between questions to allow someone who is upset to recover their composure. If someone is so upset they must excuse themselves, the discussion should move forward without them.

- **Guiding the Guide.** Sometimes an inexperienced Guide may flounder a bit in their new role. But that's okay. Other participants with more experience can always offer the Guide the benefit of that experience, and raise a hand in the meeting to clarify a point about guiding (something about discussion format or protocol, reminding the Guide of something they may have forgotten, helping them manage a participant who is challenging the guidelines, etc.). Since everyone will have a chance to take on this role, being a Guide is really a shared responsibility for everyone in the group. However, it is important that each person find their own way into a style of Guiding that works best for them, so participants should only consider "guiding the Guide" when things are getting really off-track.

- **Speaking from the depths.** Participants should take the opportunity provided after each question to look deeply into themselves for answers, trusting that there is deep wisdom within them. Then, when they speak, they should offer that insight as honestly and simply as possible, without feeling a need to explain or excuse it along the way. Sharing might be a story, an experience, an insight, or a raw emotional confession. Whatever arises in response to a question can be a powerful support to others in the group, so there is no reason to hide it away, and every reason to share it.

- **Equal time.** Everyone should be allowed equal time to share. Sometimes, especially with newly formed groups or when someone new joins an established group, one or two people can end up dominating the discussion without meaning to. Some people may find it easier to speak in a group, or hold stronger opinions about a certain topic, or feel a stronger need to make themselves heard. At these times, it is the responsibility of the Guide to remind everyone of the equal time guideline, and, if necessary, ask particularly vocal participants to allow others more of an opportunity to share. When offered in a nonjudgmental spirit of kindness, gentleness and warmth, this reminder is usually enough to help even the most talkative person become more generous.

- **Privacy.** All participants commit to keeping what they learn about each other within the group. As tempting as it might be to blog about something, or share it with a friend, or even bring it up with the person who shared after the group is over, it is very important that all participants refrain from doing this. For sharing to be honest and safe, no one should feel like they will be gossiped about or confronted after the session has concluded. Of course there would be exceptions if someone has threatened to harm themselves or someone else, or to engage in dangerous criminal activity, in which case it may become necessary to involve professional resources that can intervene or encourage participants to seek professional help. While Integral Coregroups are intended to be healing and transformative, they are not meant to become a primary resource for someone in crisis, someone on the verge of committing a crime, or someone in need of intensive personal therapy.

What about people who just don't want to follow these guidelines? At one extreme, there may be people who may want to remain silent and not participate at all. At the other extreme, perhaps there are folks who can't help being disruptive or hostile during their participation. And then there are those who just keep forgetting about one guideline or other. Since this whole process may be very new and different to people, it is important to be patient. It may take a lot of time and many gentle reminders to create an Integral Coregroup that operates smoothly. Then again, there may come a point where one person's inability to follow Integral Coregroup guidelines becomes increasingly destructive to the group as a whole. At this point, if it is the consensus of the group, it may become necessary to ask the disruptive person to leave the group if they are unable to change their behavior. A conversation with the uncooperative person should be conducted privately, quietly and compassionately, with clear expectations about what needs to change and why. Whatever the outcome, it should be for the good of everyone involved.

There are many other issues that will arise over the course of Integral Coregroups that are not addressed here, but these guidelines and definitions can get you started. For anyone interested in setting up a group, you can find additional resources at www.integrallifework.com. If you want to find a group or advertise one that you have started, those can be listed in the Integral Lifework Forum on that site. I would encourage everyone interested in caring for their inner family to participate in an Integral Coregroup, and to really stick to it for several months. The longer you are involved, the more deeply you can explore fulfilling nourishment and compassionate action in a safe and supportive community. At the same time, I would also encourage groups that have been established for a year or more to consider branching out and creating new groups with their most seasoned members – or at least to rotate new members into the group to inspire more diversity and depth.

Regular Nourishment Assessments

Another key to successful Integral Lifework practice is regularly evaluating our nourishment routines, and balancing as fairly and carefully as possible how we care for each of our inner children. One way we can do this is by reviewing each dimension of nourishment in the assessment below, and inviting others who know us well to also evaluate us in each area. For each dimension, consider how well you have nurtured your inner family in the last seven days. If you aren't immediately sure, you can always have a conversation with your inner children to find out more as described in previous chapters. I like to do this sort of self-assessment every four to six months. It doesn't matter how well I think I'm doing, for when I take a moment to inventory my self-care dimension-by-dimension, I am always surprised by what I learn. The key is to not judge myself too harshly, or have inflexible expectations about how capable or balanced I should be. Increasing our self-awareness may challenge us to heal and grow, and that is always a good thing.

So I would encourage you to make separate copies of the following page for yourself and at least three of your closest friends, family members and loved ones, and then have each person finish the entire assessment before making any comparisons.   Consider the combination of intentions, practices, habits and natural rhythms in your life that contribute to the nourishing of each inner child, and rate them using the following valuations:

   1 - Extremely dissatisfied, doing very poorly

   2 - Slightly dissatisfied or doing a bit poorly, below expectations

   3 - Satisfied, doing okay, though could still improve

   4 - Satisfied and content, meeting expectations

   5 - Extremely satisfied, doing very well, above expectations

After you have completed the exercise, take some time to compare how you rated yourself in one dimension with how other people rated you there. Did the observations of others align with how you see yourself? If not, why do you think that is the case? Did all of your kids receive similar ratings – are they in balance with each other? Are there areas you would like to improve? Remember that having one or two favorites you like to nurture most is normal and healthy...as long as other inner kids aren't being neglected or ignored. If you discover some aspect of yourself that is undernourished, consider giving it some special attention over the next week or two, providing targeted care and nurturing for that inner child. Then, if you try this assessment again at a later date, you will be able to track how your self-care changes over time.

It is often interesting and helpful to ask ourselves additional questions about our assessment results. For example, if we been giving special attention to one inner child, why is that? Have we had challenges trying to nourish a particular aspect of self, even when we try to be attentive to that dimension? If so, what types of barriers have we come up against? Do we feel confident about our abilities to parent in all areas, or are there places we struggle a bit? If we have doubts, where are those doubts coming from? Do our doubts make sense? Are the assumptions behind them true? For example, if I think I can't be a good parent to Wachiwi because I am not a physically strong or active person, how did I come to that conclusion? Am I comparing myself to others who are super athletic and highly coordinated? Has Wachiwi herself somehow communicated this to me? Or am I replaying what someone else said to me a long time ago? Am I measuring myself by realistic standards? And the same can be true of areas where I am confident, as well. Where did my confidence come from? Does it accurately reflect my abilities and talents?

It is important to remember that we may have accepted a distorted view of our own capabilities and potential without even realizing we have done so. As one example, I have a friend who helps the elderly with physical therapy. Her patients are constantly surprised by how quickly they can regain strength, coordination and even better memory and positive emotions through simple exercise routines. "I thought I was too old for this!" they will say. Well, somewhere along the line they were convinced that their age would prevent them from caring for Wachiwi or making her stronger. But this was a distortion of the truth. At the other extreme, I have counseled many couples whose idea of a successful romantic relationship was formed by watching romantic movies and TV shows about relationships. From those Hollywood versions of life, these couples developed unrealistic expectations about how easy having a satisfying romance was going to be. This created a lot of stress for them in their nurturing of Fabian, Eilon, Lada and many other inner kids, and they were perpetually feeling incomplete and unsatisfied. Very often we learn distorted, exaggerated or self-limiting things like this from our surrounding culture. But just because a lot of people believe a certain thing doesn't make it true. So part of our self-care assessment is learning how to be fair to ourselves and others – how to be realistic and accepting rather than judgmental, disappointed, overly optimistic, or frustrated.

7-Day Nourishment Assessment

	Self	Others	Total
(Wachiwi) Physical Health and Well-Being – consider diet, regular exercise, physical strength, energy, quality of sleep, chronic or recurrent illness, weight management, overall sense of well-being			
(Adelyte) Positive Emotions, Creativity and Self-Expression – consider self-expression, authenticity in communication, regular creativity and imagination, overall happiness and contentment, sense of playfulness and eagerness			
(Eilon) Relationships and Social Acceptance – consider quality of friendships and community, feeling appreciated and valued, regular expressions of love to and from other people, overall sense of connectedness and intimacy, sense of belonging			
(Manjit) Learning and Intellectual Stimulation – consider regular exposure to new ideas and opinions, excitement about learning, diversity of interests, mental alertness, overall sense of curiosity and openness, ability to think carefully and critically			
(Pemba) Accomplishment and Fulfillment – consider satisfaction over school, career, hobbies and life's work, clear sense of overall purpose, excitement about plans and goals, strength of focus, and endurance of willpower			
(Shen) Spirituality – consider the strength and consistency of connection and relationship with Inner Light, Universal Consciousness, Divine Presence, Spirit Guide(s), Soul, Spiritual Realm, Ground of All Being, Essence, or other spiritual dimension; consider ability to turn that into kindness, patience and generosity			
(Irina) Healing the Past – consider level of peace, tranquility, forgiveness and healing around any traumatic events of the past, as well as the quality of relationships with all family members in the present			
(Fabian) Legacy, Pleasure and Reproduction – consider quality of what will be left behind, frequency of pleasurable experiences, and sense of safety and stability in the home environment			
(Luceria) Ease of Shifting Between Modes of Processing – evaluate how easy it is to move from a logical, intellectual way of thinking to a felt or intuitive mode of decision-making; or from awareness grounded in the body's felt sensations and messages to analytical thought; or from any of these modes to a deeply spiritual space within; or from any mode to any other			
(Asim) Self-Concept – consider self-confidence about abilities, possession of a clear and accurate awareness about strengths and weaknesses; consider compassionate acceptance of own faults and quirks while at the same time desiring growth			
(Lada) Sexuality – consider level of satisfaction with sex life, level of genuine intimacy with self or partner, quality of physical openness, enjoyment of own body, and confidence with sexuality			
(Nobuko) Honesty and Integrity – evaluate the ability to harmonize thoughts and intentions with words, words with actions, and actions with taking responsibility for the consequences of those actions			

Additional Support

There will be times when our community of support, friends, loved ones and nourishing practices will not be enough. Perhaps after a devastating loss of a loved one we will feel confused, hurting and alone. Or maybe when we come across an upsetting memory, or information about our past that we don't understand, it will make our journey seem unbearably difficult. Sometimes we feel stuck in our journey, seemingly unable to move forward, for no obvious reason at all. And there will be times when major disruption to our personal life – some sort of crisis or really big change – halts us in our tracks. At any of these times, we should not hesitate to seek out specialized support for our journey. We need to learn how to recognize and accept our need for help, and to ask for that help without being ashamed or afraid. When I was younger, I went through some very dark times, and if I had not reached out for help, I honestly don't know if I would have survived. So I believe it is always better to seek out a community of support – and even professional care – than to "go it alone" or "tough it out." Going it alone and toughing it out are values that my family imparted to me when I was young, but they did not serve me well in times of crisis.

My hope is that, over time, more and more healthcare professionals will include Integral Lifework principles and practices in their philosophy and services, and I hope to eventually provide a list of such resources on the www.integrallifework.com website. But there are skilled, compassionate, person-centered healthcare providers everywhere. We only need to take the time to find them. The most important thing is to reach out whenever we need to, while at the same time never forgetting that we are the primary healer in the process – we ourselves hold a lion's share of the power and skill to be whole. The strength and authority to overcome challenges is there within us. We may just need someone to help us remember how to access that power, and provide us a few tools to enhance our confidence and focus. And although we will always benefit from a community of shared values that supports us in our journey, we are the navigator and captain of our own life.

However you choose to move forward, always remember that there are twelve children within you who long for your love, attention and guidance. They are also eager to reciprocate that love and affection, and, if you have cared for them in a fair and balanced way, they will always be able to support you in challenging, upsetting or depressing times. This is the joy of having strong relationships with every dimension of self: the exchange of energy, insight and loving kindness flows both ways. So this is the final and most powerful support system you can cultivate over time; a whole and harmonized self will become your most devoted friend, advocate and helper. When you skillfully care for your inner family, they can skillfully care for you. When you lavish them with love, they will always work together to make you whole, happy, thriving and well.

ADDITIONAL RESOURCES FOR INTEGRAL LIFEWORK

Print

True Love, Integral Lifework Theory & Practice, by T.Collins Logan. ISBN 978-0977033638

Web

http://www.integrallifework.com

Other

Deep Relaxation: One (An introductory audio training CD for meditation.)

www.ingramcontent.com/pod-product-compliance
Lightning Source LLC
Chambersburg PA
CBHW031319040426
42443CB00005B/136